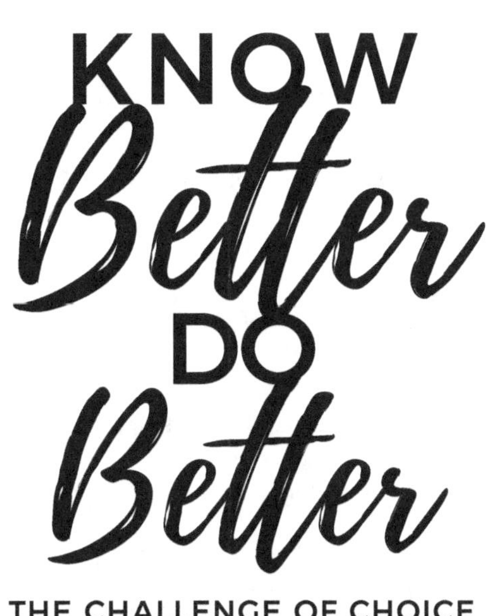

THE CHALLENGE OF CHOICE

CATRINA JACKSON

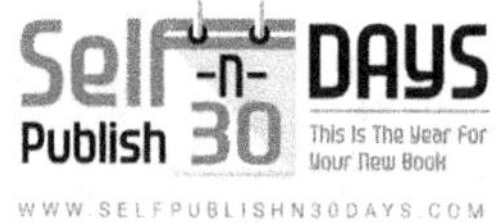

Disclaimer

The information provided in this book is designed to provide helpful information on the subjects discussed. This book is not meant to be used, nor should it be used, to diagnose or treat any medical condition. For diagnosis or treatment of any medical problem, consult your own physician. The publisher and author are not responsible for any specific health or allergy needs that may require medical supervision and are not liable for any damages or negative consequences from any treatment, action, application or preparation, to any person reading or following the information in this book. References are provided for informational purposes only and do not constitute an endorsement of any websites or other sources. Readers should be aware that the websites listed in this book may change.

Contents

Introduction

Being young and enjoying life as a young woman, I never took my health seriously. I think I was about thirty-something when my doctor first told me that my cholesterol levels were high. At the time, I really didn't understand what that meant. So, I continued living the only lifestyle I knew. As a single mom of three school-age kids with after school activities and working a full-time job, there was no time for home-cooked meals. I needed quick food, dinner-on-the-go, five nights a week. This was a vicious cycle that was on-going even on the weekend because I was so tired from running with my kids after school, working Monday through Friday, so when Saturday's and Sunday's came, we had pizza or frozen TV dinners.

Now, another year has gone by and it was time for my annual physical to follow up and check cholesterol levels again. And again, they were high, even higher than before. So alarmingly high my doctor looked at me and said, "I'm going to prescribe you medication you need to take it because your levels are over 300, which is dangerously high. You could walk out of here and fall dead". She wrote the prescription and gave it to me. As I'm driving home, I keep hearing her voice say, "You could walk out of here and fall dead." Those words played over and over again in my head. I was scared! I knew I had to make some changes. But I didn't know where to start or how to start. I knew that I did not want to take medication. I knew I did not want my body to become dependent on a chemical to be healthy (if that makes any sense at all).

Of course, I had all of the excuses as to why my levels were high, but excuses were not going to correct my cholesterol levels. It was not going away nor was it going to fix itself. That's when I decided to get really clear about what's important and get focused on changing my lifestyle. I was dealing with something that is very serious so I had to get serious! The first thing I had to do was create a balance with working full-time and my busy lifestyle. That meant I literally changed the way I thought about my life (priorities). I put into perspective what's truly important.

Originally, I started researching natural things that would help lower my cholesterol. I was so surprised when I found a wealth of information on healthy things I could incorporate into my daily life. Having done so, I am now more conscious of the things I put in my body and the things I do to my body and have a greater understanding of what having healthier habits can really do for my overall wellbeing.

That's why good health is crucial to everyone because it provides us with a sense of general wellbeing. In order to be fit and healthy, we must adopt healthy lifestyles and a proper diet. We cannot afford to be lazy. We must work hard to maintain both physical and mental health. Besides exercising, junk food should be avoided; otherwise, it will lead to obesity and health problems. It is important that we maintain optimum body weight.

Everyone needs to develop healthy and positive habits. Positive thinking helps to clear the mind and remove negative emotions and thoughts. Having positive thoughts can greatly energize and inspire us. Taking up practices like yoga can relax the mind and body, allowing room for more pleasant thoughts. Having a diet rich in vegetables and fruits can help us to become healthier and fitter. Refined foodstuffs should be avoided. One of the main reasons why we get ill is due to improper food habits, leading to diseases like diabetes and cancer. Developing a proper diet can have a profound influence on our health. Avoid picking up habits like smoking and consuming alcoholic drinks. Having regular exercise, especially in the morning, can enhance your health and leave you feeling energized throughout the day.

Taking up exercises such as swimming, biking and walking can improve your mood and health, but don't go for an activity you dislike. Doing workouts in the open air can refresh you. Do not try to change your lifestyle too drastically. Begin with simple changes and ensure that you enjoy them. Try to incorporate these simple changes into a regular habit so as to achieve long term success.

It is important for all of us to be healthy in order to have achieved happiness. Besides having regular exercise, we must have enough sleep and rest. A night of good sound sleep can leave you feeling refreshed and healthy. All these simple changes in your lifestyle can have a significant improvement in your health and wellbeing.

CHAPTER ONE

Dietary Habits and Behaviors

Why do some people always appear to get the "lucky" breaks?

What is it that makes some people successful and innately able to achieve whatever they want while others always seem to struggle?

The answers to the above questions almost always point to one reason: HABITS.

Speaking from personal experience, I made a conscious decision of being mindful that how I start my day will have a profound effect on how the rest of my day would go. From the time you wake up in the morning until when you put your head down at night to sleep, your habits mostly dictate the theme of your day, your actions and reactions and the choices you make. Before we get into explaining how and why your habits are very important in determining your success, let us first define what a habit is.

A habit is something which you do very often, and which eventually becomes an automatic and involuntary action or behavior. In other words, the majority of your most regular behavioral patterns and actions are usually done on autopilot and you are rarely even conscious that you are doing them.

So, wouldn't you agree that if you are going to do things on auto-pilot without thinking too much about them that you had better be doing the things that will most likely be beneficial for you, and which will result in

- Harmonious relationships with people

- Positive impact on the people around you

- Goals and ambitions being achieved

- Contentment, happiness, and success

The reason that your habits are so strongly lodged into your mind is because of the repetitious nature of the way they were formed. It is the same reason that you are rarely conscious of acting those habits out.

As an example, take the act of driving a car. This is undoubtedly something which we do so regularly that each of us rarely consciously even thinks about how we do it—we just do. Almost all of us have our own driving habits, such as how we hold the steering wheel or react to traffic events around us or how tolerant we are when people cut into our lane. For some people, a commute to work can be a very unpleasant experience filled with many frustrations and reactionary behavior such as shouting, aggressiveness and even dangerous driving. The stress experienced while driving is also very detrimental to the health of such people. In most cases, the individuals who react negatively while driving have been doing that for so long that it has formed into a habit. Most don't even know they are doing it.

The same applies to other habits you may have in your life such as your behaviors at work, at school, at home, around your spouse, with peers or with parents. In its own small way, every little action you choose to take in anything you do when summed up over your life determines the path that your life takes. Therefore, it is in our own best interest that we ensure that our most dominating habits are good habits which are conducive to achieving our goals.

So how do we displace existing bad habits with good habits? Below are some steps which will get you started.

How to Change Bad Habits Into Good Habits:

- Become consciously aware of your bad habits. This is the first step in dislodging them from your mind. The fact that you are reading this means that you have already begun to start this process of awareness. (Sometimes it might take a friend or spouse or child to point out our (bad) habits. If this is the case, don't react or plunge into denial but try and stay open-minded to what people are saying about you.)

- Identify ONE new habit which you would like to acquire and write it down on a pad or piece of paper. An example is: "I will listen more attentively to other people."

- Every morning when you wake up, read this habit to yourself and make a commitment that you will practice it as best you can for the whole day. Take baby steps if you need to and perhaps give yourself reminders using your phone calendar (or other electronic devices) every couple of hours or so. Do this step for at least a month because you need to allow time and repetition to firmly cement your new habit into your mind.

- After the habit in step 2 has been firmly entrenched in your mind, repeat the previous step with another (good) habit. Do these for as many habits as you wish to acquire.

The hardest thing about doing the above is committing to it and getting started. After you see the results that it will bear for you, you will be glad that you did! The main reason two people with similar opportunities in life can end up in the contrasting measures of success is based on habits. The successful person nurtured good habits while the unsuccessful person sabotaged his or her success because of some bad habits.

Many people may not even be aware that they have bad eating habits and so the question of overcoming them does not come to mind. However, these habits may seem pretty harmless when they are discussed in someone else's context; the same level of harm can apply to you as well. Going through life with bad eating habits can be damaging to your health, mental balance and even reduce your lifespan. This is the reason identifying bad habits and curbing them is very important for improving your lifestyle to a healthier, sustainable one.

BAD EATING HABITS INCLUDE:

1. Overeating, which means ignoring the messages from a satiated stomach and continuing mindlessly to eat one bite after another, is the top bad eating habit. This kind of behavior is usually linked with a problem of self-discipline, whereas the person cannot correctly interpret intense hunger pangs and may have tried to curb them unsuccessfully before succumbing to a binge eating session. The

root cause of overeating must be eliminated so the activity of eating is pleasurable and allows one to chew slowly, savoring each morsel and slowly feeling full in order to maintain eating regular portions.

2. Affinity to junk food may well be a matter of convenience for most individuals addicted to stuff easily available through a phone-ordering service, internet ordering, front door delivery, or simply by poking your head out of the car in a drive-through restaurant. In small measures, it is not harmful, but mammoth portions and daily dependence on junk food leads to eating out of boredom.

3. Speed eating may have been cute when you were five, but it's time you realized that mealtimes are not competition time for outdoing yourself (or others) in gobbling down your food! Usually, it is stress that causes people to turn into speed eaters.

4. Going Vegas-style on the weekend after a week's worth of controlled eating is no better than a binge attack from displaced discipline. It is an inappropriate reward system and completely monopolizes sensible eating.

Hydrating Properly

What to drink and what not to drink to stay hydrated. Water is the best fluid you can drink. You need to drink between six and eight cups of water a day. Water is natural, has no calories, and will replenish your body better than any other fluid on earth. The primary value of hydration is to keep your body functioning the way it is designed to function. Your muscle tissue is made up of approximately 75% water.

When a car engine runs low on water and you keep driving the car, the engine will overheat, parts will start to fail and eventually, the car engine will stop working. When you deplete the water in your body your muscles will cramp, you will become tired and your body will start to shut down some secondary systems so that the basic systems can operate. If you stay dehydrated for too long, your body will become violently ill and eventually, you will die from a lack of water.

- Sports drinks can help to replace electrolytes that you have lost, but you need to be careful with these beverages. Many sports drinks are loaded with sugars and other ingredients that you do not need. Search for sports drinks that are low in sugar and sodium.

- Stay away from caffeinated beverages.

- Try not to drink anything with alcohol in it because alcohol actually dehydrates you.

Ways to Keep you Properly Hydrated

- Make it a goal to drink between seven and ten ounces of fluid for every twenty minutes of exercise you do.

- Drink sports drinks and coconut water each day to help replace electrolytes.

- You can get some of your fluids by eating fruits that will provide you with fluid and natural electrolytes.

- Sometimes you may think you are hungry when actually ; you only need to drink water.

- When you notice a decline in energy and feel fatigued, then drink more fluids.

Eating Healthier Meals

Eating healthy is a matter of picking foods that aren't processed and eating foods that are closest to their natural state as possible. Foods such as fruits and vegetables have natural vitamins, minerals, and sugars that are good for your body. Fruits will satisfy your sweet tooth and give you loads of vitamins and minerals and add natural fiber to your diet. Fresh vegetables will give you a wide variety of vitamins and minerals too, and they should be steamed to retain their natural value. You should watch what toppings or sauces you put on your vegetables because they can be the source of added calories. Avoid processed products and try to stick to whole grains for pasta or baked goods as a healthier alternative.

When looking for your meat fix, go for lean meats and don't forget the fish. Sometimes we lack omega-3 polyunsaturated fatty acids that are present in naturally grown fish. Instead of frying the fish, you can grill or bake your fish because that is a much healthier choice.

When looking at other meats, bison or venison may be healthier than beef which will have a higher fat content. Although foods like lunch-meats, hot dogs, bacon and sausages are cheap and convenient, they have saturated fats and they also contain unhealthy preservatives. There are healthier alternatives to these processed foods, make sure you ask for them at your local grocery or find them at health food stores like Whole Foods.

When you eat a variety of whole foods, you allow yourself greater intake of the vitamins and minerals needed to live a healthy life. Mix up the meals and make sure you are getting the basics like dairy products, fresh fruits and vegetables. Stick to natural beverages instead of soda or artificial juices. Drink water, milk, or 100% fruit and vegetable juices. Limit the sugary soft drinks to a bare minimum. Everyone wants a little taste in their beverages from time to time and water doesn't always satisfy those needs. Adding a slice of lemon or touch of flavor powder is a healthier alternative to those sugary soft drinks.

Reasons for Eating Healthier

Some, if not most, people who try living healthy are concerned about making changes in their meal schedule. Even with the fact that eating healthier meals has a lot of benefits to bring. If you are not convinced to eat healthy foods yet, here are seven reasons for eating healthier:

LOSE WEIGHT

Eating healthy will help you lose weight. Replacing unhealthy foods with healthy ones will definitely trim down your calorie count. Eat white meat, fruits and vegetables instead of candy and juices. Instead of getting fat and toxins in your body, you get vitamins, minerals and fiber instead. Taking junk food and sodas completely out of your daily diet will result in losing two to three pounds a week without any exercise.

LOWER THE RISK OF CARDIOVASCULAR DISEASE

Taking in unhealthy fat, such as saturated fat, animal fat and certain dairy products, is a primary contributor to getting heart disease. With a diet of healthier foods, executed with a meal schedule and less fat, there would be fewer risks leading to coronary heart disease and stroke, which is primarily caused by atherosclerosis—the narrowing of the arteries.

INCREASE ENERGY

Junk food and other alternative snacks may give you energy, but it can never compare to the energy given by healthy food. Most of the time, what junk food gives is a dash of energy that lasts for a short period of time. It is known as the 'sugar rush.' With a balanced and healthy meal, you will have enough energy that will last the whole day.

INCREASE STRENGTH

Healthy foods not only give an ample amount of energy but also strength and endurance. Healthy meals give enough nutrients to nourish the muscles, bones and other parts of the body for strenuous and prolonged activities.

LESSEN BOWEL AND DIGESTIVE PROBLEMS

Problems in the digestive system and the intestines often result from low intake of essential fiber that can be found in a healthy and balanced meal. Eating healthy will lessen the possibility of getting constipation and help regulate bowel movements.

LOWER CANCER RISK

Some cancers are caused by smoking, alcohol consumption, processed foods, high-fat foods and smoked foods. When choosing to eat healthily, these things should be kept to a minimum, if not completely taken away from one's lifestyle, thus lessening the risks of cancer.

IMPROVE REST

Yes, eating healthy foods can give you a peaceful sleep. The balanced amount of carbohydrates and protein found in a healthy diet helps the body adjust to the changing levels of energy when sleeping. And therefore, a full-rested and energized feeling is guaranteed upon waking up in the morning.

Eating healthier improves not only your fitness but also your emotional state as well. With this, you are bound to have a healthier body and project self-confidence and self-respect that comes along with it.

A Few Healthy Eating Tactics

There are more than a few tactics that help with healthy eating. But a few of my favorite tactics for good dietary behavior are:

HEALTHIER DESSERTS

If you are like me, you crave a little gourmet sweet, even when you are trying to eat a healthy diet! You will ask yourself, "Can I indulge in desserts on a special family dinner night and it's still considered healthy?"

As a general guideline, we all need to avoid sugar, but eating desserts in moderation is acceptable for a healthy diet. Let's not forget that a healthy diet is a lifestyle and not a temporary situation, so we should be able to enjoy our food while abiding by some good nutrition rules. Moderation and balanced nutrition are really the key elements for a healthy diet. But when it comes to selecting that special dessert, is sugar the only enemy to avoid? Here are some guidelines that I use to select the ideal dessert for my family dinner.

If you are buying your dessert:

- Go for all-natural ingredients or, if possible, look for organic products.

- Avoid desserts that have trans-fat and hydrogenated or partially hydrogenated oil.

- High fructose corn syrup is bad for you. Recent studies have shown that consumption of high fructose corn syrup leads to excessive accumulation of fat compared to the same consumed amounts of regular sugar.

- Avoid artificial coloring and all sorts of fancy name preservatives. Read the labels: if you cannot understand what that ingredient is, it is most likely not natural and not good for you.

If possible, make the dessert from scratch with all-natural ingredients. It will be guaranteed healthier for you and it will taste better too! While selecting the right recipe, go for light desserts, with reduced fat and reduced sugar. Unless advised by a doctor for a specific medical condition, do not substitute butter for the less healthy margarine alternative, or sugar for artificial sweeteners, just try to use a recipe that uses less of these ingredients and uses low-fat milk products.

AVOID MARGARINE

Margarine is bad for you because it is high in trans fatty acids, which increases cholesterol. Margarines are made from a vegetable oil base of polyunsaturated fats. These fats must go through hydrogenation, a chemical process used to increase the melting point of the product. Soybeans, corn, cottonseed or canola seeds, oils extracted by high temperature and pressure. The remaining fraction of oils removed with hexane and other solvents. Oils, now rancid, steam cleaned to remove all vitamins and antioxidants, but pesticides and solvents remain. Oils mixed with a nickel catalyst, Oils with catalyst subjected to hydrogen gas in high-pressure, high-temperature reactor. Soap like emulsifier mixed in, then oil steam cleaned again to remove horrible odor. The gray color is removed by bleaching. Then artificial flavors, synthetic vitamins and natural color added. The mixture is packaged in blocks or tubs, advertised and promoted as a health product *(PreventDisease.com)*.

AVOID ARTIFICIAL SWEETENERS

Also known as nonnutritive sweeteners. These began with the need for cost and caloric reduction. It is interesting to know that artificial sweeteners were actually chemicals being developed for another purpose when the researcher tasted it and found it was sweet. Since the 1950s, nonnutritive sweeteners have allowed us to have our sweets without the calories and cavities. There are five nonnutritive sweeteners approved by the FDA. There has been great controversy since 1997 about the health consequences of ingesting these products:

- Saccharine
- Aspartame
- Sucralose
- Acesulfame
- Neotame

H.J. Roberts, MD reports that by 1998, some of these products were the cause of 80% of complaints to the FDA, symptoms include: headache, dizziness, vomiting, memory loss, seizures/convulsions, and fatigue. Along with these symptoms, links to aspartame are fibromyalgia symptoms, numbness in legs, joint pain, anxiety attacks, sclerosis, systemic lupus and various cancers. *(MedicineNet.com)* Use natural sweeteners like dates, agave, maple syrup, and even bananas they are good for you and they taste better!

In your quest for that special light and healthy gourmet recipe, keep in mind that calories matter, but they are just part of the story. Healthy, natural ingredients are good for your body. For example, keep in mind that, although more calorie-rich, nuts in general, and especially walnuts, which are mainly used in European recipes, contain very beneficial omega-3 fatty acids that are healthy for your body and brain.

More good news: recent research shows that chocolate is actually good for you! Dark chocolate (at least 70% cocoa) contains a significant amount of antioxidants that are very beneficial for your body. Try not to combine it with milk, though, as this is shown to reduce the body's capability to absorb the antioxidants.

REDUCE CALORIES

Losing weight can be a challenge for many people. Most have tried various diets and exercise plans only to find that they gain everything back again plus more when they stop.

The only way to lose weight long term is to reduce and substitute the types of calories that you are consuming and to add exercise on a regular basis. The number one rule to determine if a diet is healthy and lasting is by asking yourself one simple question, "If I had to, could I eat this way for the rest of my life and be healthy?"

If the answer is no, which is the case with most fad diets, then chances are the diet you're considering would cause you to lose more than just a few pounds of extra weight. Diets that exclude certain food groups, or come with crazy rules, like only eat plain, baked potatoes with nothing on them for a week, then only drink apple juice for three days ... and so on can cause serious vitamin deficiencies.

People who already struggle with low iron or other vitamins and minerals could find these diets are permanently damaging to their bodies. It is a better idea to change unhealthy eating habits and practice calorie substitution. This way, your body is still getting the nutrients and calories it needs to be healthy and efficient.

Substituting fatty foods for leaner foods also helps you keep your metabolism working at its maximum efficiency. Diets that require you to starve yourself cause your body to go into storage mode and everything you eat turns to fat. This is part of the reason why when you come off these diets, you gain a ton of weight.

There are a few simple tricks that you can learn to help you be successful long-term. Cutting back on calories will make a big difference; also regulating the type of calories you are consuming will change your health for the better.

The first thing to do is commit to permanently eating less. Keep a journal for a week or so, record everything you consume from a glass of water to pizza, and even a stick of gum. You will be surprised what you are consuming throughout the day and where those calories are coming from; the results can often be alarming.

Start simple by consuming smaller portions. Eat slowly, giving your stomach time to tell you it's full. You will still need to eat enough to be able to function and have energy, so plan when and how you will accomplish this. Remember, calories translate to energy.

There are empty calories that come from sugary foods. They give your body short bursts of energy. However, there are whole calories that come from foods like vegetables, which also provide energy, but the energy is prolonged. Foods that have carbohydrates like bread will also give you a sustained feeling of fullness. The trick is to eat these in moderation.

There are several common misconceptions about eating schedules. For instance, some dieters only have two meals a day and do not eat after 6 p.m. or another set time. The truth is, rules like these will vary depending on lifestyle, genetics and schedules. If you are going to bed at 8 p.m. then yes, eating before 6 is a good idea.

Those who only eat two meals a day often end up eating twice as many calories as they should because by the time they eat, they are starving and they don't recognize when their body tells them it's had enough. Not to mention, most of those calories end up being stored because the body thinks it's not getting fed enough.

Eating less has been shown in studies to help reverse aging for people who want to stay young and healthy longer and can be easy. It might mean that you must eat more frequently to sustain the type of energy level your body needs. Or it might mean eating bigger meals earlier in the day, and a smaller meal in the evening.

Your body must deal with the food that comes in and this can be stressful if there is too much or too little. For some people, eating several small meals throughout the day can mean less calorie consumption. But for others, it can mean more. It is about finding something that works best for you and your lifestyle.

Eating fewer calories can be as simple as substituting your afternoon candy bar for a granola bar or drinking water 20 minutes before your meal or at the beginning of your meal. Water has zero calories and will take up space in your stomach, helping you to feel like eating less.

Eat the foods that are high in fiber first. Fiber also has zero calories and will help you feel satisfied as it takes the body longer to process these foods. This is an easy thing to change since there is plenty of fiber in vegetables.

Then, when you eat the rest of your meal, you won't be as hungry and will be less likely to eat as much of the fatty meats, white-flour pasta, or dairy products, which have zero fiber.

Save your leftovers for another meal. Reducing calories like this can be a lot of fun if you are willing to be a little creative and flexible. You may not see drastic overnight results, but the results that you get will stick. There is no point in losing weight if you are only going to gain it all back after you finish your diet, and the yo-yo dieting can cause major health issues.

CHAPTER TWO

Physical Activity Habits and Behaviors

In my personal journey, I found being physical is just as equally important as my dietary lifestyle. Physical wellness is essential for your overall fitness level. It encourages you to apply principles of good health and knowledge which will positively influence any habitual bad patterns you may have.

Consider Your Physical Wellness

Physical wellness involves respecting your body's own uniqueness and diversity as well as engaging in practices that move you towards a higher level of health. Optimal physical well-being includes connecting with your physical self and avoiding harmful habits while remaining focused on the balance of body-mind-spirit.

There are four major factors to consider when trying to assess your level of physical wellness:

Physical Fitness

This includes maintaining appropriate cardiovascular conditioning, muscular strength, muscular endurance, flexibility, and body composition. By this, I don't mean you necessarily need to be at the gym every day of the week. In fact, you don't need to be at the gym at all. Anyone who follows me on social media knows how big I am on home workouts. It's much more inexpensive and effective than going to the gym.

Nutrition and Balanced Diet

This means practicing healthy nutrition and a balanced diet that consists primarily of fruits and vegetables with a few seeds and nuts.

Self-Care

This includes being more aware of your body. Meaning, you should be able to notice within the next second any unusual changes to your body regarding your thoughts and emotions. The practice of daily meditation will do wonders for you in helping to calm your mind and attain more peace in your life.

Respect Where You Live

By this, I am not referring to the regular upkeep of your house. It involves practicing overall environmental upkeep. It is as simple as becoming more aware of not littering. Take care of the Earth, which takes care of you. By practicing a simple act such as not littering, you become naturally filled with genuine joy. This resonates with intrinsic feelings that you have shared a part in improving your community.

So why is it important to develop your physical wellness? There is ample evidence indicating that adopting a lifestyle that supports physical wellness has benefits related to:

- Maintaining good health
- Increasing your level of productiveness
- Prolonging your longevity

This goes a long way in helping you to naturally and gradually reduce any personal and societal health care costs which you may have, ultimately improving the quality of your life.

Keys to Remember

Stay Physically Well. Nurture your mind, body, and soul.

Mind

Your mind needs intellectual stimulation for growth and challenge. Practice being able to gather emotional strength through self-acceptance and improving your self-image. Be more positive.

Body

Your body gains strength through physical activity and exercise. If you challenge yourself physically, your body changes and evolves positively. This then allows you to naturally become healthy and able to meet the demands of your day.

Soul

The spirit within you helps give you purpose in life and assists in motivating you to personal growth. Spirituality guides you to be more respectful to people, and to display moral and ethical behavior.

Squeezing Physical Activity into Your Schedule

We all know that exercise is good for us and we've all heard that exercising is the healthiest thing to do. You might feel reluctant about exercise thinking that you'll need to join a gym or buy expensive equipment but in fact, physical activity can be done at a very low cost or no cost at all. Maybe you relate exercise to jogging or any other kind of exercise you dislike, but you need to change your way of thinking. You can gradually incorporate physical activity into your life and make it fun.

It might be very challenging for people who have many pounds to lose. If you are suffering from obesity, you might feel uncomfortable exercising around others not being able to bend or move around as easily as they can. Or, you might think exercise will harm you and sure you can do it, but there is a safe way to get physically active. You don't have to join a fitness center and you can start moving at your own pace right at home. Inactivity is risky and you can hurt your body even more by not exercising.

Don't be Scared of Exercising

Physical activity doesn't need to be a highly-disciplined effort. Start adding activity a little at a time throughout your day. Be active at home while doing your house cleaning, try walking with a friend, raking leaves, mowing the lawn, just be imaginative and find ways that will get you moving more. Exercise to a work-out video or dance! Just find something you will enjoy and make sure you feel comfortable with the activities you choose.

Set Yourself up to Succeed

If you want to stay motivated, try adding variety to your physical activities and make sure you exercise on a regular basis. Just like any other habit you incorporate into your life, you need to make exercise a part of your daily routine. Other ways to spark your motivation include:

- Start by setting up short-term goals that are achievable

- Plan ahead and be creative

- For extra encouragement, exercise with a friend

- Exercise to music and make it fun

- Find an exercise that you can manage and that fits in with your schedule

- Track your progress and don't forget to reward yourself when you achieve.

If you put your mind on being active and focus on improving your health, you will succeed. Just knowing that exercise will improve your health can be a great motivator to keep you physically active. For most beginners, the hardest part is to get started. Remember, exercise does not need to be strenuous and it should not be something you dread, so pick an activity that you will enjoy. You can benefit from moderate exercise if you make it a regular, permanent habit that will become part of your life.

Choose an exercise that will be appropriate for you. If you can't accomplish an activity the first time, don't put yourself down. Don't be too hard on yourself and start at a level you can manage by working your way up slowly, especially if you have been inactive for a long time. Allow yourself time to develop the skills you need for an activity to become enjoyable. As your body gets stronger and you become fit, you can then increase your activities to keep them more challenging.

Start by increasing the amount of time you spend doing an activity. For instance, if you start walking 10 minutes a day on your first week, gradually lengthen your walks to 15 minutes the following week. Eventually, you can start walking faster and increase your walks to 18 minutes.

If you want to gain health benefits, you sho're alluld engage in moderate physical activity for at least 30 minutes per day. If able to do it all at once, just break them down into three 10-minute workouts throughout your day. If you can stick to your physical activities for at least one month, you will be on your way to making exercise a regular, permanent habit. Being physically active will make you feel great, more energetic and once you start experiencing the health benefits of exercise, you won't want to stop.

Workout Motivation

How do we find the motivation to exercise? At the end of the day when that big fluffy couch seems to be calling your name and nothing looks more appealing, what is it that keeps us on track and motivated?

In order for me to teach you how to motivate YOU, I have to share how I motivate myself. Everyone is different and everyone needs motivation served to them on a different platter. What motivates one doesn't necessarily motivate the next. Some people need constant encouragement. Others need a kick in the ass. Some need to be told specifically what to do. I personally, like so many others, need the challenge and the goal. For years it was easy for me when I was roller skating. It was a good form of cardio and I skated to stay fit and lean. Now, I have to find other ways to keep myself motivated and, trust me, I know sometimes it's hard.

There are literally hundreds of different ways to motivate yourself to exercise and I will give you a few examples of what has worked for me. I sometimes struggle to keep going but the most effective way to keep motivated for me is having a workout partner. Having that buddy on the same page as you, challenging you to push hard and keep going always motivates me. Writing down my program and keeping track of it is also a great method for me. I track my results and, week by week, I check to see my improvements. What better motivation is there than seeing results?

Caloric expenditure is one that has worked for me in the past as well. I know that you read tons of weight loss articles and they say don't count calories. Well, how are you going to get the proper amount of calories you need and burn the proper amount without keeping track? Knowing what I need to burn in the day pushes me that extra little bit or keeps me on track so I don't expend too much.

Simple enjoyment from exercise and having fun will keep anyone going. I wish I could workout with everyone; I would train all day every day. If it wasn't for the fact that it takes away my concentration on the individual, I would love to work out with them all. Having fun doing a group or boot camp class has always been motivating for me. Lately, I have been riding my new mountain bike and I love it. Doing something that keeps you moving while you are having fun can't be bad for you.

Internet articles, blogs, books any type of information and reading material are interesting for me and get me to try new things or methods and different exercises. Sometimes reading what others have done and their success stories are very inspirational.

Set goals and when you reach them, reward yourself. It's always nice to get to a goal and it's even nicer to know that you are getting something for your hard work. I like to get some sort of little reward for every goal I achieve. Set your goals and set your rewards and get them often.

Keeping my "favorite pair of jeans that are a little tight" around makes me work hard to fit into them and want to look good. With looking good comes feeling good and having those outfits I feel stellar; it keeps me on track.

Stress relief is a great motivator for me. Some days I need to blow off some steam and putting on my favorite workout jams on my iPod while I'm just tearing it up at home really clears my mind and drains the stress from my body and mind.

Clearing my head while riding my bike has worked great as well. Again, it's a stress relief that really gives me time to think about other things and maybe just take in some scenery.

In the past, having a coach or a trainer around to push me helped wonders. I always tell my clients that I love to have a personal trainer for motivation.

I like to keep pictures around of myself. Seeing myself lets me know that the healthy, hard-working girl is still in there and it is possible to be like that again. Also taking before pictures motivates me to get to my goal. Nothing feels better than looking in the mirror and seeing yourself in great shape and comparing it to where you were.

A couple of other motivators that may work for you could be signing up for a 5K or 10K race, not feeling bad from missing workouts, extending your life expectancy and being able to run and play with your grandkids. Weighing yourself and keeping measurements could also offer you motivation. Do not do these things every day but once a week. Trust me, as you see the numbers going down you will be motivated.

However you choose to motivate yourself, whether it be from taking those measurements, logging your workouts or reading motivational quotes, the feeling you get once you have reached a goal and people are noticing is priceless. Make and set your goals so they are achievable and realistic. You will reach them as long as you work at it and there is no better reward than feeling great and looking great and having others notice.

Maximize Your Workout Results

Modern life is hectic, no one has enough time, there are a gazillion things demanding your attention and since fitness isn't your profession or your first love, it's the gym time that ends up suffering.

This is only natural. We're forever promising ourselves that we'll do an extra-long session next time just as soon as we've finished with this budget/school/holiday/deal. Little and often, however, is a much better way to exercise than sporadic blitzing. For a start, it means you're less likely to half-cripple yourself by launching an under-prepared body into an overambitious workout. It's also easier mentally to keep up the momentum and the feel-good factor, since mega sessions with long gaps in between quickly become daunting and may lead eventually to canceled gym memberships. This makes it easier to monitor progress—a motivational bonus—plus frequent short spells in the gym will do more to raise your metabolism on a daily basis than the once-a-fortnight gut-wrenching osteopath special.

So how can you make sure you get a decent workout when you only have a few precious minutes to dedicate to the temple of toning?

Try the following:

HAVE YOUR KIT READY, PACKED UP, AND BY THE DOOR

Einstein used to line up seven sets of clothes on the hangers each week so he never wasted precious brainpower deciding what to wear or trying to find it. Take his lead. When you pull stuff out of the dryer, match it up into complete sets of kit, then make sure you have a gym bag ready to go for every day. Leave it sitting by the door like a patient dog hoping to go walking and it will be both convenient to grab and a helpful reminder to your conscience.

PLAN YOUR WORKOUT, WORK OUT YOUR PLAN

Nobody has enough time at the gym so who are all those people wandering around from cardio room to weights and back? Be clear in advance what your workout goals are. Don't fix on a single machine—it may be in use—but decide in advance how much cardio you're going to do or what weight session you have in mind.

TRY GOING EARLY

What? Like in the morning, working out before the day gets its claws into you means you start out feeling good and get your metabolism up and running. There are also fewer people and it's hard not to feel virtuous which makes you more likely you'll be back tomorrow.

TRAIN WITH YOUR BELOVED/KIDS/FRIEND/CO-WORKER

Don't force fitness to compete with friendships and love life—not a good idea; you will become a sad individual. See if you can mix gym/social life by training with friends and family. This may mean thinking a little laterally. You may have trouble getting your spouse to show up to an abs class, for example, but swap it for something more fun like a core class and you can frolic with the whole family.

DON'T REST, CROSS-TRAIN

Your gym tells you to spend no more than 20 minutes on a machine? Fine, just leap straight off it and onto another one. Take ten on each if you like. Forty minutes working on a mix of rower/treadmill/bike will give you a more thorough workout than the same time spent plodding away at the same machine. It uses different muscles and psychologically allows you to put more effort because you know you are changing soon.

DON'T REST, SUPERSET

Normal practice if you're doing weights is to rest at least 30 seconds in between sets. Well, don't. Instead, switch straight to an exercise that works the opposite set of muscles and cut to and from between the two with no rest time at all. For example, if you're working biceps, then alternate with a triceps press. Pair chest press exercises with lateral pulldowns. Hamstrings with quads, etc.

Miscellaneous Physical Activity Habits

People that engage in physical activity are healthier than ones who don't. When you walk into a building, is your first thought to take the stairs or the elevator? There are far more benefits that come from being physically active than not physically active.

When you engage in exercise and physical activity, you reduce your stress level and increase your energy. Make sure you exercise on a regular basis to keep your stress low and your energy high.

There is a natural remedy for depression that many people do not talk about. That remedy is exercise. There are many details that go into this, but doctors have found exercise is a natural cure for depression. On a side note, you will increase your self-confidence and well-being when you exercise.

When you stay physically active, you will manage your weight much better than being physically inactive. You will have a lot more stamina and energy throughout your day. You will also have a decrease in back, neck, and shoulder pain when you start staying physically active on a daily basis.

Your quality of sleep will surely improve when you stay active and exercise during the day. Your alertness will be much keener and you will live a lot longer with a much more satisfying life.

You will have a lot more mental creativity when you stay active. During brainstorming sessions, this will come in handy and it is when you will truly notice the difference in your mental creativity.

Your sexual life will become much more fulfilling and inspiring when you stay physically mobile and take care of yourself.

When you stay physically active, you will have a more positive outlook on life. You will be more optimistic in nature, causing you to enjoy life much more than you would have otherwise. You will become much more productive from getting exercise a regular basis. This productivity will carry into all areas of life, especially while you are at work.

There have been many stories where people who get on a regular exercise routine and stay active end up dropping some medications they were once on. You will need to check with your doctor before getting off any medications that you were once taking; doing this without doctors' orders can be very damaging to your health. Exercising also encourages other healthy habits that you will naturally move towards, such as eating healthier foods.

CHAPTER THREE

Lifestyle Habits and Behaviors

The concept of metabolism in weight loss is one that, when effectively harnessed, can help a lot of dieters lose weight in a very healthy and sustainable manner. This prevents resorting to quick weight loss solutions, which experience has shown only have temporary weight loss benefits.

While metabolism does play an important role in an individual's overall weight loss ability, it is equally important to understand that it is something that can also be affected either negatively or positively by lifestyle habits. Therefore, besides genetic and hereditary factors, your overall lifestyle choices and actions have a lot to do with your metabolism.

Metabolism can, therefore, be said to be one piece of the weight loss puzzle that can be effectively increased by modifying and making the right lifestyle choices.

Lifestyle Habits

Below are some of the lifestyle habits that can positively impact and increase your body's overall metabolism.

EATING A HEALTHY WELL-BALANCED DIET

It is no mystery that what you eat and how you eat it does affect your metabolism and mood. The resultant effect of either makes you feel energetic or lethargic. Therefore, it is advisable to eat many small, well-balanced meals (about 4–6) in the course of your day and also control your calorie intake. This is arguably one of the fastest ways to increase your metabolism.

ENGAGING IN REGULAR EXERCISE

Aerobic and strength exercises can perhaps be said to be the fastest ways to dramatically increase your overall metabolism. The harder you exercise during your aerobic and weight training workouts, the more you will be strengthening your cardiovascular system by supplying more oxygen to your body cells to burn more fat for energy while also building more lean muscles which are very metabolically active.

SLEEPING MORE

Lack of adequate sleep (both having trouble sleeping and not getting enough sleep) can negatively affect your overall metabolic rate as this deprives your body of the repair opportunity and energy replenishment which having adequate sleep provides. Therefore, aim to get 7–8 hours of sleep each night.

RELAXING MORE

Try to avoid any form of emotional or physical stress as they stimulate the body to increase its level of stress hormones, particularly cortisol and adrenaline. These hormones are catabolic (destructive metabolism) in nature and are associated with premature aging and cardiovascular diseases and generally make it difficult for the body to build muscle or strength.

DRINKING MORE WATER

Water not only serves as a great appetite suppressant, but also helps to boost digestion by improving the emptying of the stomach and intestines while also reducing gas, bloating, and constipation. Water also helps to purify the system by flushing out sodium and toxins from the body. Ensure to drink about eight glasses of water daily to get the best results from this natural weight loss elixir.

GIVING UP EXCESSIVE ALCOHOL AND SMOKING

You should realize that a lot of alcoholic beverages are filled with calories just as much as most sugary soft drinks. Studies have also shown that drinking alcohol during meals actually encourages over-eating. Equally, a cigarette contains nicotine, which like its stimulant counterpart caffeine, is known to temporarily increase metabolism but has far greater negative side effects than benefits.

Conclusively, understanding that metabolism plays a very important role in achieving and sustaining healthy long-term weight loss, it would, therefore, seem logical to try to incorporate or improve on these positive lifestyle habits in order to significantly increase your body's metabolism and to boost overall your fat-burning ability.

IMPROVE YOUR SLEEP HABITS

Stress is one of the problems that has caused a lot of people sleepless nights. Those people experiencing sleeplessness may have a sleeping disorder, sleep deprivation or insomnia. One of the most typical sleep aids for them to take is over-the-counter or prescription sleeping pills. Unfortunately, those medications often have negative side effects. There are, however, some all-natural alternatives.

Chamomile tea, standardized Valerian, Skullcap and Melatonin are some of the herbal insomnia remedies that are natural. Those natural and drug-free sleeping aids are very helpful and effective to improve your sleep into a deeper stage. For example, the standardized Valerian can ease your nerves, and by drinking chamomile tea with melatonin, your mind and body can be calmed and relaxed, which can help you to fall asleep easily and quickly.

Besides using natural sleep remedies as your sleep aids to help you improve your sleep, you also need to focus your sleep habits and sleep hygiene. By having a good and healthy daily diet, right emotional levels, good habits, and correct sleep routine you can greatly improve your sleep at night.

Exposure to natural sunlight during the day, especially early in the morning after the sun just rises or late evening before sunset for at least 30 minutes to 1 hour, can improve your sleep too. You can walk, stroll or do some exercises outside your house in the garden to make yourself tired. The more tired you are, the easier and quicker you can fall asleep at night. Natural sleep assistants should help you attain a deep sleep quickly and easily, which can really improve your sleep effectiveness. How do you know that you have effectively improved your sleep? You will be able to easily and quickly fall asleep waking up in the morning feeling refresh and energized.

MANAGE YOUR STRESS

When you are in the middle of a stressful situation, you may find yourself making unhealthy choices and poor decisions. These choices can negatively affect both your professional and personal life. Therefore, it is crucial to learn stress management techniques to avoid such mistakes.

Understanding and Managing Your Stress

A clear, collected mind is the most effective way to keep a handle on your stress levels. One particularly good way of staying calm in the face of stressful situations is to sit down with a pen and paper (or blank computer document, if you prefer), and identify in writing the actual causes of your stress. Then, make a list of the options you have to tackle each one. Don't try to take them all on in one sitting, it'll be overwhelming, and in the end, more stressful for you. Instead, look at only one stressor at a time and focus on how you have the power to work towards eliminating it.

There are many different ways to learn about stress management, and some will work for you better than others. It's best to consult a variety of sources to find which is best for you. You can hire a stress management consultant, take a class, or speak with a friend or colleague who is particularly skilled at it. You can also find a lot of reading materials online or at a bookstore. If you choose to go online, in addition to articles and e-books, you can find forums with stress management experts who can answer your questions about dealing with personal, professional, and romantic stress (among many other kinds).

A Few Ideas to Get You Started

If you're just beginning to work towards managing your stress, you may be inundated with options. Give yourself time to master each technique, and in the meantime, try these short-term fixes to quickly decrease your stress:

MASSAGE

These are great to help decrease your stress and one could say "a nice way to pamper oneself." Relaxing massages vary in lengths and price ranges, depending on your free time and economic situation.

- **Swedish massage** is a gentle type of full body massage, great for tension, and for those who are sensitive to touch.

- **Deep tissue** is used for chronic pain and if you have a lot of muscle tension.

- **Hot stone massage** helps ease muscle tension, promote relaxation and relieve stress.

- **Shiatsu** is thought to be the most relaxing, promotes emotional and physical calmness, helps relieve headaches, depression and anxiety.

AROMATHERAPY

Nature has provided us with essential oils that are derived from plants, flowers, herbs and trees with medicinal aromas can have an amazing effect on one's emotional and physical wellbeing just to name a few:

- **Rosemary oil** is activating, it improves your overall mode with effects of alertness and competency.

- **Peppermint oil** improves digestion, acid reflux, nausea/morning sickness, makes you feel invigorated.

- **Lavender oil** is calming and relaxing, good for insomnia, restless leg syndrome, it also helps with hot flashes.

- **Frankincense oil** can help you overcome allergies, sinus infections and sore throats.

Aromatherapy can be incorporated into a massage, or you can purchase your own essential oils or incense from a health food or New Age store.

Use them in your home or office. Soon, these scents will become associated with relaxation and will help you reduce stress when you smell them.

MUSIC

Don't ignore the soothing power of music! Hearing your favorite songs, or listening to calming melodies, can help distract you and remind you of happier, less stressful times.

- Make yourself a playlist or mix CD of songs for study time, it puts you in a good state of mind, helps to improve memory.

- Listening to music can improve your mood and make you feel happier.

- Working out to your favorite playlist can really boost your physical performance.

Moderation & Balancing Your Lifestyle

As technology advances, so does western medicine and the position of many people on alternative healing methods, there is little dispute that a daily multivitamin is beneficial to our overall health and wellness. People are showing increased general interest in maintaining a more appropriate diet and of the ways that they're keeping the balance without making drastic diet changes are through the daily multivitamin.

In general, a solid daily multivitamin and/or mineral supplement will improve your overall function and boost both the physical and mental wellbeing overall. This is because the multivitamin will improve the function and circulation of your organs. As circulation improves and the tissues receive the vital nutrients delivered from the multivitamin, they begin working at a highly efficient state.

If you couple that with improved diet and exercise programs, not only is the body achieving a greater state of wellness but the improved circulation and function of the organs (including the endocrine system) will help to improve mental function.

That may seem out of reach for people that have had an impaired function for so long, but when we live the traditional western lifestyle it can be expected that we grow used to the state that we're in. It's like growing accustomed to an unpleasant odor. After a while, the feeling of fatigue, lack of focus and poor motivation (general melancholy attitudes overall) all become second nature and we get used to it. Once you start to take a daily multivitamin and pair it with even something as simple as a daily walk, you'll begin to feel the positive effects almost instantly.

- Improved energy

- Greater focus

- Better memory retention

- Improved breathing

- More peaceful slumber

While this isn't an immediate change (vitamins aren't an instant cure-all), they will help to gradually improve your overall state of wellness and should be treated exactly as intended; a daily multivitamin supplement—to help supplement your improved diet and exercise plan.

If you want to balance your body, there are a number of things that can be done. One strategy that you can use to balance your body is to change your diet by eliminating unhealthy foods that are high in saturated fats and sodium and instead concentrate on consuming foods that are healthier such as fruits, vegetables, and whole-grain foods.

Another strategy that can help you achieve optimal health is exercise or some sort of consistent physical activity, which will effectively help reduce stress. Eliminating the stress in your life, whether it be through exercise, yoga, meditation, or any other solution, can reduce acid levels and help balance your body. Balancing your body can help prevent sickness and can help your natural healing process become more effective.

An excellent way to help you achieve optimal health and enhance your body's pH and natural healing abilities is to drink pure alkaline, antioxidant-enriched water, also known as ionized water. It can be a highly effective resource to help neutralize much of the excess acid your body produces, as well as help to reduce acid build-up from years of an unhealthy lifestyle.

Burnout

Burnout is a serious risk when you are not able to balance your work and your personal life properly. It is comprised of mental and physical exhaustion that can be experienced in relation to stress in your working environment and lack of proper management. When your personal life and work are in harmony, the chances of burning out are very slim, giving you a mental safety net for juggling between those aspects of your life.

In our world today, most adults are expected to hold a job and bring in the money in order to maintain their family's lifestyle. They also have their own career goals to meet, which means having to work on a daily basis. On top of that, they are expected to spend quality time with their children and be a good partner to their significant other. Overall, they have many expectations to live up to in their day-to-day life.

When both partners are working every day, there needs to be a lot of compromising and adjusting to maintain a relatively sane lifestyle. It is usually understood that whenever possible, free time should be quality time with the family. There are times, however, when problems crop up with the family. This usually means that work is sacrificed in order to sort out whatever difficulties there are. In the meantime, the work that is being left behind is piling up. Therefore, when the time comes that the person is finally able to deal with it, he usually finds the workload to be far too much. This results in working late nights, trying to do everything and be everywhere at once. In this case, family time is now being sacrificed. It is in these situations that the stress becomes too much and the person ends up burned out.

Avoiding burnout is not as difficult as some make it seem. Achieving the right work-life balance is really about managing your time and your life better. Once you make this decision to employ proper time management and self-management, you are on your way to getting that balance that you are searching for.

The most necessary step is to admit that you need help. At the very least, open up to someone and admit that you are finding it hard to close the gap. Nearly everyone has gone through this type of situation in one way or another, which makes it easier for him or her to understand. There are many unexpected and difficult situations that arise, and most of the time things do not go as planned. In times like these, you need to open up and explain your situation and your inability to cope. In fact, after explaining your side, you could even ask for advice on how to deal with it better.

You also need to give yourself some "Me Time." This means focusing on your needs, keeping track of how you are feeling and all that. After all, you cannot really take care of others properly if you, yourself are in dire need of some TLC. To sum it all up, it is important to be more aware of yourself. If you are drained at the end of the day, day after day, then you already know that you need to do something about it. Steps to take include talking with your partner, asking for some help, and if possible, minimizing your number of tasks. Another option, although not realistic for many, would be to look for a less stressful job. In the end, you must do what is required in order to manage your life better.

CHAPTER FOUR

Mental Health Habits and Behaviors

Health is a very important part of human life and plays a crucial role in the development of human beings, the revolution of society, the updating of culture, and the change of lifestyle. However, what is the definition of health? Health not only means no disease of the body, but also emphasizes mental health. How to keep a healthy body and mind? The following tips will give you a reference.

First, set clear goals in life. We pursue a lot of things during our life. However, due to living environment, social culture, and individual condition, we cannot make all our dreams come true. And this requires us to set goals for the limitation of one's time and energy. In order to realize the value of life and pursue larger development in a limited time, it is better to make sure what you want and set clear goals. With a clear goal, you can effectively eliminate all kinds of negative emotions and keep vitality to challenge.

Second, keep a forgiving attitude towards others. Nowadays, competition among people is fierce for advanced science and technology. Clear goals and success in life are certainly key elements to keep healthy. However, leniency and corporate progress also benefit to one's happiness and health. Sometimes, you will get unexpected results by helping others selflessly.

Third, develop good living habits. Good habits can make a contribution to people for a lifetime. We cannot underestimate its value to health. But in real life, many people ignore this important aspect. Those people keep bad habits in life. For example, some people like to spend all night playing cards or watching TV, which will do serious harm to health. According to scientific research, the activities of the human body are controlled by the biological clock. The violation of it will cause the disorder of body function. So, we should keep good habits in all aspects of life to ensure the best function of the entire body system.

Fourth, ensure there is enough exercise in your life. It is proven that physical activities can keep a clear mind and nimble though. Because exercises can enable appropriate rest for the brain to maintain its workability and promote the blood circulation to improve the function of the heart. Moreover, sports can adjust a person's psychology to keep vitality. Regularly exercises can also improve a person's adaptability and strengthen the resistance to disease, then to live a healthier and longer life.

In addition to these, reasonable nutrition composition and essential hobbies are also in favor of physical and mental health. In order to live an easy and happy life, please draw attention to the maintenance of your health.

Does Mental Health Affect Physical Health?

The effect of positive or negative emotions is so powerful, it changes lives. It is widely documented that a person's emotional health influences medical outcomes and can lead to depression or happiness.

Research shows that one function of the human brain is to produce substances that affect emotional and physical health. One such substance is endorphins which play a vital role in the body's ability to heal itself. These studies show that laughter can reduce stress, decrease pain, lower blood pressure, and boost the immune system because laughter increases endorphins which increase immune function and make you more resistant to disease.

Do you ever wonder why you feel better after a good laugh, a long run, having sex or any strenuous workout? It's because of the endorphins released in your body which gives an elated feeling that sometimes lasts up to 14 hours depending on the individual.

What are Endorphins?

An endorphin is one in a group of opiate-like peptides produced naturally by the body in the brain at neural synapses. At various points in the central nervous system pathways, they modulate the transmission of pain perceptions. The term endorphin was derived by combining the words "endogenous" and "morphine." Endorphins produce a morphine effect to increase the pain threshold, produce euphoria and sedation. This effect can be blocked by naloxone which is a narcotic antagonist medication.

Endorphins may also regulate the release of growth hormones from the pituitary gland and are released when you, for example, cut your finger or burn your hand. Initially, you feel severe pain but it soon disappears due to the release of endorphins that kills the pain.

HOW TO RAISE ENDORPHIN LEVELS?

Most of it could be prevented with more attention to healthy habits, thoughts, emotions, nutrition, and actions. How do you respond to stress in your life? Any prolonged strenuous exercises such as swimming, walking, bike riding, cross-country skiing, tennis, having sex will raise endorphin levels, "the happy juice." UV light increases endorphins but even with the risk of getting skin cancer, people still sunbathe. People will continue to be out in the sun because it leads to that "euphoric feeling" and people like feeling good. Laughter is good medicine for the soul and it raises endorphins levels. Keep laughing!

It's time to start taking big steps towards creating that balanced life you want. Just as endorphins increased your happiness and outlook on life, positive attitude and thoughts increased your mental health. Set big financial goals, start a successful home-based business so you can make the money needed for a healthy financial future. Eat healthy foods with the right portions to prevent weight gain and obesity. Exercise frequently to reduce stress, increase circulation, maintain desirable body weight and have a belief system—prayer works! Remember your mind or body is a terrible thing to waste.

It is now generally recognized that difficulties of training, poor habits, school problems, temper tantrums, enuresis, and childhood delinquencies are evidence of emotional disturbance which may be corrected by proper investigation and treatment.

Feeble-mindedness is an incurable congenital deficiency with a strong hereditary basis and, as such has little relation to mental or emotional disorders. It is primarily a problem of eugenics and sociology.

Even such an incomplete listing of psychiatric problems forces us to recognize that we can no longer regard mental illness or insanity as the only field for psychiatric investigation. Emotional disturbances and personality problems, which may be regarded as lesser forms of mental illness, constitute ever-present problems, touching all of us.

Theory of Mental Illness

From the scientific data at hand, we have no reason to conclude that heredity is a major factor in the causation of mental illnesses. In spite of this, heredity is commonly believed to be their most important cause. This belief is unfortunate, for the assumption that mental illness is caused by heredity leads to the conclusion that it cannot be prevented or cured.

To assume that mental illness is hereditary because it "runs in the family" is erroneous, because it is impossible to separate the effects of the environment, or so-called "social heredity," from those of physical heredity. By social heredity is meant the transference of traits of character or types of behavior by contact with an imitation of those persons with whom one lives, while physical heredity implies the transmission of characteristics or types of behavior through the reproductive cells.

One has only to consider the abnormal environment which exists in a family in which there is a mentally ill person to realize the great possibility of a child in such a family becoming mentally unbalanced, even though no hereditary factors are active at all. In order to establish the hereditary character of a disease, one must demonstrate that the disease was not caused by environmental factors and that it follows recognized laws of inheritance. Neither of these requirements has been met in the case of most mental diseases.

Furthermore, it does not follow that, even if a hereditary factor were present, the development of the disease could not be avoided by the manipulation of environmental factors. Hence, we should turn our attention from the heredity theory of mental illness to what may be more profitable approaches.

Certain mental illnesses have a definite physical basis. For example, the psychoses of general paresis, arteriosclerosis, senility, injury, brain tumor, etc., are due directly to the destruction of brain tissue.

Furthermore, delinquency, hallucinations, fears, compulsions, or other emotional disorders may be due to disturbances in the functioning of the glands of internal secretion; to infectious processes, the toxins of which give rise to states of delirium; the action of drugs; or to the actual destruction of brain tissue. Such conditions may, and do, give rise to strange thinking and behavior. Their prevention and cure are problems of physical health, just as are the prevention and cure of any other physical disease.

On the other hand, ideas and emotional attitudes are more often a product of the social environment than of the physical disease. A man may let his hair grow to shoulder length because his thinking has been deranged by the activity of the spirochete of syphilis in the cortex of his brain, or he may wear his hair long because he has been taught a religious belief in which long hair is worn as a symbol of the Christ-like life. In the first case, we explain and treat his unusual behavior on a physical basis. In the second, we explain it in psychological and social terms.

In the investigation and treatment of the abnormal behavior and thinking which constitute the material of poor mental health, it is necessary both to investigate those physical disturbances which may interfere with the complex functions of behavior and belief and to recognize those factors in the environment which may disturb these same functions. There is no real dichotomy or conflict in these approaches. In some cases, physical disturbances predominate, while in others, mental and social situations are of major importance.

I firmly believe that the whole universe is interconnected. Our body, mind, and spirit are deeply rooted in each other. If the body is sick, the mind cannot relax or feel good. And if the mind is not relaxed, it will give birth to stress and that will lead to chronic health problems.

So clearly, in order to possess a sound body, we must have a calm and peaceful mind. Without a sound mind, we cannot expect our potential growth or development.

Personal Habits and Behaviors for Happiness

Most of us have taken our health for granted; it is imperative that we begin to make it a priority in our lives. Today, people are dying way too young due to unhealthy lifestyles and many others have been prescribed numerous medications just to cope. The pharmaceutical companies are getting richer, but our health is deteriorating at an alarming rate because our bodies are not meant to process the chemicals that are being put into it through drugs. In order for us to get our health in order, we must implement some changes that will help us get to the health condition we desire. Here are lists of changes that will help us stay on task to better overall health.

EATING PROPERLY

The body functions properly when it is nourished with the right foods. Many people are so busy that their daily diet consists of unhealthy food from fast food facilities, this is not good. Because this has been the case, obesity has risen and continues to rise each year. We must make better choices when it comes to the food we eat. Reading labels and preparing our own meals will go a long way in changing this around for our good.

By far the most twisted information ever spread through the mass media is the information on what food you should put into your body. Special interest groups for meat, milk, corn, orange juice, every possible food group, all with good intentions, deliver a message that distracts you from the basics of healthy eating. Special diets for different diseases—hypoglycemia, high cholesterol, diabetes, heart disease, cancer, obesity, and the list is almost endless are too often too 'special,' and only replace one health problem with a new health problem.

EATING PROPERLY IS EASY

You can find powerful food sources that you can easily incorporate into your lifestyle, but if convenience is an absolute necessity, you can eat properly even from easily accessible food restaurants. The main staples of your diet can be found easily in these places, and in common restaurants, but you need to learn what foods are the best for you at each of these restaurants.

EATING PROPERLY IS DELICIOUS

Food that is excellent for you and your health is far more satisfying to your palate than the typical, disease-causing food you are probably feeding yourself every day. The sickening, disease-causing foods are normally the consequence of a craving. Explore the sources of your cravings and how to extinguish them, easily and painlessly. You will discover how only brief periods of eating delicious, healthy foods will make you crave delicious, healthy foods.

EATING PROPERLY BRINGS INSTANT RESULTS

Eating well will bring you, instantly, greater energy, greater confidence, a greater immune system, and a stronger sense of well-being. Eating well constantly will allow you to have these qualities constantly. Discover the amazing difference between a good meal and the meal you may be used to, the difference in how they make you feel, and even how they make you behave.

A diet that is proper will reduce more disease than any of the 'special' diets do. Once you understand the basics of a pure, pristine means of eating you will understand how much myth and folklore you have been fed about what to eat and how to eat.

Incorporate a supplementation program to add to your daily diet. Understand how the body works and what supplements are most effective for you. A nutrition pyramid, beginning with the basics such as vitamins, minerals, and essential fatty acids, is a good way to start on the path to better health.

We must take control of our health and commit to maintaining a healthy, strong body for many years to come. Take the proper steps that will lead you to your desired result. Manage your stress, give up smoking, and eat properly for longer life and a healthy one.

CHAPTER FIVE
Fitness Habits

Have those extra pounds been sneaking onto your body through the years, without you even being aware of it? Has your conscience been dropping hints that, hey, you've got do something?

So what's the problem? Or is it excuses? I don't have time. I don't feel motivated, and it's too late to make a difference. These are just some of the reasons I've heard. So many studies have now proven the many benefits of getting off the couch and making a dedicated effort to change your fitness mindset. Just a twice a week bicycle ride or a long walk will do wonders for your self-esteem and start a gradual weight loss. It could be as simple as leaving the car at home and riding your bicycle to that restaurant you go to for breakfast on Saturday morning. If that's too far, find one closer to you. Just riding through the quiet residential streets near you, waving at people tending their lawn makes for a pleasant start to your day.

Whatever you start out with, don't try to do too much too soon. That's a sure recipe for burnout. Just a walk around the block will do.

Keeping motivated will be difficult at times but knowing why you want to make a change will keep you on track. If you find yourself falling off the wagon at times, forgive yourself and get back on track. It really helps to make it fun, with little rewards along the way. When you lose five pounds, reward yourself with buying something you wanted, or that movie you wanted to see. Starting a journal could do wonders for you, such as keeping track of your goals, jotting down what you ate and what you did every day to reach them.

The ugly fact about workout programs is that most people drop them. That does not make the person or the program a failure; it often takes a few tries before finding a workout that sticks or learning enough about yourself that you can make anything stick. Current research on building good health habits shows that it takes two months of repetition tied to a behavioral trigger before a habit becomes maximally automatic, much longer than conventional wisdom suggests. Making fitness a habit requires more than forcing yourself to go to the gym every day for two weeks. Making fitness a habit requires longer and more intentional repetition and a strategy to condition your mind. So, consider the following four keys to building good habits and sticking to your workouts will be much easier and your fitness success will be much more achievable.

Increasing Your Success

Your chances of success in forming any habit go up as the amount of repetition, simplicity, triggering, and consistency goes up.

REPETITION

Intend to repeat the action at least every day. Multiple times a day is better. Research shows that missing a very occasional day does not affect the rate of habit establishment, so don't kick yourself if you slip up. But research also shows that more missed workouts equal less habit-forming so intend to repeat at least every day.

SIMPLICITY

Simple actions become habits much more easily. Actions like "grab the pull-up bar" and "do a push-up" will become habits much more easily than "begin my 7-device workout circuit" or "change clothes, find the DVD, and follow Jillian for 15 minutes." If you can establish the more complex workouts as a habit, that is great! Those workouts are great. Complex workouts just do not easily become a habit for most of us, so when you are having trouble making a habit, make it simple.

TRIGGERING

Strong habits are triggered by daily actions that you would perform anyway. Pair a habit you want with a habit you already have. Simple and high-repetition trigger pairs such as "press START on the microwave → reach up for the pull-up bar" and "take off my shoes → do a push-up" work much better than "remember to drive by the gym on the way home on Tuesdays and Fridays."

CONSISTENCY

Every time you do the trigger, do the habit you want to build. The more you do it every time, the more it becomes a habit. That is a big reason why simple actions with frequent triggers "stick" more often than complex workouts on infrequent schedules.

Family Fitness, Including the Children

As a parent, you are aware that you set an example for your children, good or bad. If you get involved in fitness training, you can be showing yet one more example to your children.

Your example as a parent is one of the most powerful tools a parent has. If you show them how exercising changes your health and attitude, they just might be pulled into wanting to workout also. Your children are curious creatures and will be drawn to new experiences, especially if they see it has a positive effect on you. With this, the power of suggestion goes a long way.

The same goes if you are taking part in poor health and nutrition choices. If you observe the people when you are out shopping or hanging out and you see a parent-child family around, at least 90% of the time if the parents are overweight, the children are too. Again, children are curious about what mom and/or dad are doing. They learn from their parents and imitate them.

You have the power to influence how healthy your family will be. The younger your children are, the easier it will be to encourage them to get started on a fitness plan. It will be even easier if you work out with them but watch out how you work out because they may want to imitate EVERYTHING you do. Fitness habits started early have a better chance of staying with them. It will be the best gift you could ever give your children.

The best thing is you do not have to TELL your children to exercise with you. You may want to invite them but wait until they start watching you as if they are curious. Just start working out for yourself, and workout in the living room or someplace that gets a lot of traffic from the kids. The chances are great that your child will just want to try it. Curiosity will pull them in.

Why is Fitness So Important to Our Overall Health?

Many people hated having to take gym class when they were in school, but there is a reason that physical fitness is emphasized so early. In addition to the side benefits of fitness, exercise is necessary for someone who hopes to live a long and healthy life. If someone does not know why fitness is so important to our overall health, they should consider the physical and emotional benefits of a good workout.

Obviously, the most important reason to exercise is to avoid becoming obese. Most people realize that obesity can cause many serious health problems, such as heart disease, stroke, diabetes, high blood pressure, and cholesterol. What they may not realize is that it can also lead to problems such as sleep apnea, arthritis, and even infertility. Rather than dealing with these serious issues as they arise, avoid them by practicing good fitness habits.

When someone is not feeling good about themselves, they reflect that feeling to everyone around them. Exercising on a regular basis is a great way for someone to improve their self-esteem. They will not only look better, but they will be proud of themselves for taking control of their condition. This feeling will be obvious to everyone and it will help someone improve both their personal and professional relationships.

When someone is not getting the right amount of exercise, they may be distracted by their concerns about their health, but that might not be the only reason they cannot concentrate. Exercise increases blood flow to the brain. When someone exercises on a regular basis, they will notice that they are thinking much sharper than before and that they are better able to concentrate on tasks.

Many people who work out on a regular basis talk about a "runner's high" and there is actually some truth to what they are saying. Exercise releases chemicals in the brain that make it easy for someone to relax and feel happier. If someone is dealing with a lot of stress or unhappiness, exercising is an excellent way for them to clear their mind and unwind.

People who do not know why fitness is so important to our overall health will be surprised at how much better they feel when they start working out. They will not only lose weight and become physically healthier, but their mood will improve. Everyone should be able to find time in their schedule for some exercise that will significantly improve their overall quality of life.

Taking regular exercise has many health benefits that will not only make you feel good but also make you look younger. Exercising regularly will help to increase your cardiovascular strength which is very important for your health.

If you want to lose weight and gain more energy then you should consider taking more exercise and make it a part of your day. If time is scarce then you do not have to do it every day as you will benefit if you can exercise 3 or 4 times a week. It does not mean that you have to exercise for long. For example, exercising for as little as 15 minutes a day can have enormous benefits. It also means just being more physically active by getting your butt off that couch and start moving.

Regular exercise has many health and preventative benefits as follows:

REDUCING THE RISK OF CANCER

There have been many studies that have concluded that there is persuasive evidence that people who take regular exercise reduce their risk of getting cancer. This is especially true with cancer that has hormonal element ssuch as breast cancer in females and prostate cancer in males. People who exercise regularly tend to have lower incidences of these cancers. Another form is colon cancer which medical research has revealed that exercising on a regular basis can also reduce the risk.

DIABETES PREVENTION

By taking more exercise and being more physically active you can decrease your risk of diabetes. Medical Research into people who are more physically active lessen their chances of developing diabetes. (Colberg, et al., 2010)

HEALTHY BODY WEIGHT

A healthy body and weight go hand in hand. People who are physically active burn more calories and achieve a more balanced body weight throughout their lives. Maintaining your natural body weight helps with preserving lean muscles and improves the effectiveness and efficiency of the body's functions and movements.

MIND AND BODY

Keeping active has emotional and physical benefits. Medical studies have revealed that exercising more and just being more active has positive effects on reducing anxiety and depression. It can also help to reduce stress and tension that is so common these days. Exercise releases the body's feel-good chemical serotonin. Good exercises that are can keep you fit and healthy as well as relaxed are yoga or Tai Chi. Combining stretching poses, movement and deep breathing will help you relax in the mind and body.

CHAPTER SIX

Breakfast

If your house was anything like mine when my kids lived at home when they were younger, then you know how chaotic mornings can be with school-age kids. In the mornings, everyone in my house would be scattering to find either their backpacks, schoolbooks or the car keys. Out the door, you go!

What about breakfast? Don't worry I will get something later at school/work. Does this sound familiar? 99% of households around the world wake up in this fashion and leave the house without having any breakfast.

"Breakfast is the most important meal of the day" is an old saying that everyone knows, but hardly anyone follows. Yes, exercise is important for athletic development, but that all starts with having breakfast.

Why is breakfast so important?

From an early age, there is no doubt that you will have been told that you should always make sure that you eat breakfast, as it is the most vital meal for us all. But why is breakfast the most important meal of the day? This is something that I am going to explain to you, as well as attempting to highlight why breakfast doesn't take much time to prepare and is not of inconvenience at the start of your day.

Is breakfast the most important meal of the day, really?

Yes, there is no doubt that breakfast is the meal of the day that you should not be skipping, especially if you are on any sort of diet. This may sound strange because it is never going to be anyone's main meal of the day, as this is generally going to be lunch or your evening meal.

The fact is that breakfast is critical to fuel your body for the day ahead, or at least for the morning that lies between you and your next meal. Without it, you are not going to be as awake or alert, and there is much more chance that you are going to end up snacking due to hunger creeping up on you. By starting the day with a small meal, you are doing a better job at waking yourself up, you are giving yourself the energy you need to carry out your daily tasks, and you are making sure that your hunger is suppressed for long.

After fasting through the night, your body has shut down and needs rebooting, which is exactly what the consumption of food first thing in the morning does. It is also true that what you put into your body at this time of the day will affect how it performs.

What are the Best Things to Eat for Breakfast?

So, what should you eat for breakfast? This is a very good question, and here are some important examples, accompanied by explanations as to why they should play a part at breakfast time.

Fruit

You should be eating at least five different portions of fruit and vegetables every single day without fail. By starting off the day with at least one of these you are giving yourself a good head start to achieving what should be a very manageable goal. How much time does it take to eat an apple, orange or banana, or some pineapple chunks? An apple or a banana, for example, can be eaten on the way to work, so no excuses that you don't have time. Fruit is packed with nutrients that your body needs, sugar to provide you with energy and fiber to help keep your hunger satisfied. What's more is that there are not many calories found in fruit, making them appealing to everybody.

Wholegrain cereal

This is amazingly nutritious and loaded with fiber that will help to suppress your hunger. You can get huge amounts of minerals such as iron from eating muesli and granola, amongst loads of other essential vitamins and minerals. You can add some chopped fruit to it to make it tastier (another portion of your five a day), or also a sprinkling of sugar to give yourself an added energy boost. Multigrain Cheerios are also another popular cereal that you should take into consideration, low in calories and crammed full of nutrients.

Cereal takes about 30 seconds to prepare, so again it is hardly slaving in the kitchen to prepare and taking up valuable time in the morning.

Eggs

Eggs are full of protein and can be eaten in a variety of different ways including boiled, fried, poached, scrambled; and this is likely to be the most time-consuming effort at breakfast time. They are nutritious and as long as you are not eating several at a time they are not going to send your cholesterol levels through the roof. They also go well with other aspects of breakfast such as some whole-meal toast.

You can even make a hard-boiled egg the night before and leave it in the fridge to eat in the morning, saving you some more time.

Grab a drink too

A cup of coffee is a great pick me up in the morning; its caffeine content will undoubtedly help wake you up. Water is also going to be a great calorie option to wash down what you are eating. There is also the fruit juice option such as orange juice, apple juice or cranberry juice to name a few. These are highly nutritious and will, if nothing else, give you a mega-dose of vitamin C. Even a glass of cold milk is going to be a nutritious option for a drink first thing in the morning, low-fat or fat-free is even better if you are on a diet.

Healthy Recipe Ideas

If you really don't know what to have for breakfast, or you are really unsure as to what is going to be healthy, and what isn't, get yourself a cheap breakfast cookbook, have a look on YouTube for a free video guide on healthy breakfast recipes, or follow some food blogs online. There is so much free information on the internet that all you need to do is make time for breakfast, decide what to have, and determine what is good for you!

IT DOESN'T NEED TO TAKE AGES TO PREPARE

So a bowl of cereal, some fruit you can eat on the move, an egg you have prepared the night before, and the time it takes for the kettle to boil to make a cup of coffee, are you really putting yourself out making time for breakfast in the morning? If you really understand why breakfast is the most important meal of the day, and how it can do nothing but good for you, then you are going to know it is worth making time for, even if that is just ten or fifteen minutes before you dash off to work or school.

WHY IS MAKING SURE YOU EAT AN EXTRA MEAL GOOD FOR THOSE ON A DIET?

So, is making sure you eat an extra meal is a good idea for those on a diet trying to eat less? Yes, as breakfast is the most important meal of the day that is exactly right. If you eat right in the morning then you are going to be doing any diet that you are in the world of good. If nothing else it will be because you are ensuring that you don't go hungry the whole morning and end up snacking on something that may not necessarily be diet savvy. It is easy to get yourself a low-calorie breakfast full of nutrition that is going to do your body all sorts of favors at the start of the day. It is down to you to make the change to your routine to ensure that you do this every single day, though. Get to bed and get up fifteen minutes earlier. Whatever it takes to give yourself a bit of time in the morning to get something to eat, you have to do it.

DON'T HAVE THE SAME THING EVERY DAY

Definitely switch it up, variety is key, that way you will end up sticking to a routine to have breakfast each and every day of your life. If you eat exactly the same thing every day then you are only going to end up getting bored with it. Have toast and cereal one day, and fruit and eggs another. Whatever it takes to make it more interesting and appealing will help to ensure that you don't slip back into bad habits and start missing it again. If you really want to be sporadic then write several breakfast meal ideas down and put them in a hat, draw one out each day so you can prepare as much as you can before you go to bed the night before, saving you valuable sleep minutes in the morning!

So now you know why breakfast is the most important meal of the day, and how it is easy to prepare in a very short space of time, there is no excuse for you not to make that lifestyle change starting tomorrow morning.

LOSE FAT BY EATING A HEALTHY BREAKFAST EVERY MORNING

From as far back as I can remember, my mother pounded two things in my head that are still with me today. They were to "always wear clean underwear" and "eat a healthy breakfast every morning." The first one does not require anything more to be said. But eating breakfast every morning is something many people just don't understand as important.

The most common excuse is there just is not enough time to have a healthy breakfast every morning. Most people settle for a bowl of sugary cereal, a portion of fast food drive through, or worse yet, they skip breakfast all together.

Why is breakfast important? You must fuel your body every morning with a healthy meal. If you wait until lunchtime or a mid-morning snack, your metabolism starts to shut down, and your body now starts to automatically store fat for energy and starts to burn lean muscle mass just to keep going. This is known as starvation mode. You need a healthy breakfast every morning to jump-start your metabolism.

Eating a healthy breakfast every morning does not need to be a time consuming and elaborate process. Including preparation time, you can make a healthy breakfast in less than 3 minutes. This breakfast consists of the following:

- Quaker Oatmeal Weight Control

- One sliced medium-size banana

- Half cup of almond/coconut milk

Microwave a packet of oatmeal for 1 minute with 2/3 cup of water. Slice up the banana, then add the almond milk. In total, this delicious meal has only 314 calories, a whopping 12.2 grams of protein, and a measly 3.6 grams of fat. Compare that to an Egg McMuffin or your favorite Starbucks coffee.

So, take a few minutes and do something good for yourself. You will be amazed at how in just a few short weeks eating breakfast just like the one described above every morning, you will start to notice positive changes in your body.

CHAPTER SEVEN
Vegetables and Fruits

Are you one of those people who hate vegetables? No matter how hard you try you just can't seem to choke down spinach, broccoli or brussels sprouts. You know vegetables are good for you. They are packed with vitamins and minerals, but you just can't stand the taste. You may be part of the 25% of the population with a specific gene that makes you especially sensitive to bitter and pungent flavors. WebMD classifies people with this genetic characteristic as "supertasters." Whether you are a supertaster, or you never liked the flavor of any vegetable, there are ways to prepare them so that they are delicious. Try including vegetables to help you enjoy eating healthier foods.

Creatively Including Vegetables

Here are some suggested tips to include vegetables:

MASK THE FLAVOR WITH CHEESE

Cheese dishes are a tasty way to mask the flavor of vegetables.

For example:

- Lasagna and casserole fans can add healthy vegetables, such as zucchini, broccoli or cauliflower, to your favorite dish.

- Layer some thin slices of zucchini into baked lasagna. The flavor of the cheeses and sauce masks the natural flavor of the zucchini.

- Steamed broccoli added to macaroni and cheese will give you all the nutrients and none of the natural bitter flavor of broccoli alone.

- Try adding some chopped bell peppers, a few bits of chopped onion and a slice of tomato to a cheese omelet.

If you are counting calories, use a low-calorie, low-fat cheese.

ADD VEGETABLES TO SOUP

Try adding a few fresh carrots, peas, corn and potatoes to your favorite soup, such as chicken noodle soup. Add carrots to most any flavorful bean soup. French onion soup is a rich, pungent soup that lends itself well to adding a few potatoes. Keep some bags of frozen vegetables in the freezer. Add a few spoonfuls to a can of ready-to-eat soups like cream of mushroom or cream of chicken and simmer until the vegetables are tender.

TRY YOUR LEAST FAVORITE VEGETABLE IN A SALAD

Raw vegetables are especially healthy. Cooking can remove many vitamins and minerals, but over-cooking vegetables can destroy nutrients. Slice your least favorite vegetable thin and slip a few slices into your salad. Mix lettuce with a few spinach leaves and some finely shredded cabbage or carrots. A flavorful vinaigrette dressing will mask the flavor of most vegetables without adding a lot of extra calories.

ADD VEGETABLES TO SPICY FOODS

Finely chop mushrooms, zucchini, eggplant or broccoli and stir them into your spaghetti sauce. Simmer until the vegetables are tender and then serve the vegetable spaghetti sauce over a big plate of whole wheat pasta. You can even add some finely chopped carrots or some whole kernel corn to the sauce. The spices and tomato base used in spaghetti sauce will cover the taste and the vegetables will add interesting textures to the sauce. Add some thin slices of zucchini or eggplant to a spicy pizza and bake it as you normally would.

JUICE VEGETABLES

Add fresh vegetables to your favorite juice drink. Use a juice machine or a blender to juice some carrots, beets, cucumbers, an apple, and some broccoli. Strain the pulp and add it to a glass of orange juice. You won't taste the vegetables, but you will get plenty of valuable vitamins and minerals. Any vegetable can be juiced with fruits and blended with your favorite fruit juice. Vegetables can be taken in any form, be it juices, salads or plain boiled; but always ensure that they are washed carefully before consumption to avoid complications.

The Importance of Vegetables in Weight Loss Programs

It is an unfortunate fact that most of us take the view that vegetables are rather unpalatable. This is a shame because if you are trying to get rid of some weight by shedding fat, vegetables are your best friend. The more vegetables you can include in your diet, the more effective you will be in your weight loss endeavors. So, if you don't already do so, do try to make a point of increasing your vegetable intake.

You should take note that vegetables are packed full of nutrients and minerals essential for the support of life. On the other hand, they do not contain very much in the way of fats and sugars. So, they contain, in general, the kind of things you want to take in when slimming, and not so much of the things that you do not want to take in.

You can eat, leafy, green vegetables, without limit. Vegetables such as kale, sprouts, cabbage, carrots and the like are all very good for you and again, you can consume as much as you like. However, having said that, I must point out that it is no good smothering your salad with loads of mayonnaise, coleslaw, salad cream or similar. If you want some form of accompaniment, try to keep it to something without too many calories attached.

Make it a regular thing to eat green leafy vegetables once a day. At least eat a large green salad, and include mustard, cabbage, lettuce, radish, tomato, spinach, and any other salad leaves. Also, you need to include vegetables containing a lot of water, such as celery and cucumber, because they add very few extra calories, at the same time, help to keep you hydrated.

The only vegetables that you need to eat in limited quantities are those that contain a lot of starch. These basically are root vegetables such as potatoes, beetroot, parsnip, sweet potatoes, yams, etc. Remember that these vegetables are mostly composed of carbohydrates and will add a lot of calories if consumed in large quantities. Just a few portions of starch-rich vegetables, per week, should be enough, and it is preferable to eat them in the earlier part of the day. This way your digestive system gets a chance to break the food down before you get into bed.

Raw foods are generally best when trying to lose weight and this is particularly true of vegetables. However, we all know that there are some vegetables that you cannot eat raw, like most root vegetables and some brassica. In this case, they are best cooked by steaming in preference to boiling since boiling removes some of the nutrients and minerals in significant amounts. Preferably, you should not fry vegetables, because this increases the calorific content considerably.

Advantages of Frozen Vegetables

Fresh vegetables are some of the healthiest food you (and your kids) can eat, but many people don't realize that frozen vegetables are just as good for you and sometimes even better. Because of this, they are often written off from the shopping list, but this is a mistake even if you prefer fresh vegetables. There will always be times when frozen vegetables should make their way into your diet. Let's look at the three primary advantages of them.

ADVANTAGE 1: FROZEN VEGETABLES ARE NUTRITIONALLY SOUND

- Freezing acts as a preservative for vegetables so there are no chemical additives required that serve no nutritional benefit or possibly even harm the vegetables. The freezing process inhibits the growth of bacteria and other particles.

- Canned vegetables, on the other hand, add salt as a preservative and inhibitor. Sometimes many other useless ingredients are also added. Too much sodium and other stuff in the diet can lead to adverse health effects like high blood pressure.

- While it seems to be conventional wisdom that frozen vegetables are better for you than canned vegetables, many people think that they are less optimal for your health than fresh vegetables. While this can be this case sometimes, it is not true most of the time. Based on a 1998 report from the FDA, frozen vegetables have the same amount of health benefits and nutrients as fresh vegetables.

Freshly picked vegetables from a garden or farm that are picked at their peak ripening period may the best health-wise, but rarely do you find these types of vegetables at the grocery store. Often, they are instead picked prior to fully ripening so they won't be overripe at the store, and in this process, they lose some of their nutrients. Frozen vegetables, on the other hand, can be picked at their optimal ripening time and then quickly frozen to retain their nutrients.

ADVANTAGE 2: THE CONVENIENCE FACTOR

Frozen vegetables are simple to prepare, especially when compared to fresh vegetables. With fresh vegetables, you must clean them, peel them and cut them. With frozen ones all you need to do is place them in the cooking container—there is no prior processing needed.

If you have little time for preparing dinner, who wants to take the time to process fresh vegetables? Chances are you will skip them, and if that's done enough your health won't be optimal. Frozen vegetables are a great substitute for fresh ones when time is a factor.

ADVANTAGE 3: IT IS EASY TO MIX YOUR FLAVORS

Frozen vegetables are also often available in mixed packages, already chopped and diced in ready-to-eat condition. Or you could buy individual packages and mix them yourself easily. If you are making homemade soup, mixed frozen vegetables are a quick and easy way to add nutrition and taste to your recipe.

Feel like having broccoli mixed with corn and carrots? You can simply buy a bag of that at the store, but imagine having to prepare that with fresh vegetables? You would have to wash and chop the broccoli, husk and scrape the corn off the cob, and peel and dice the carrots. You would be lucky to prepare that dish in less than an hour. With a frozen package, you could be eating this mix in five minutes. So, if you enjoy the rainbow of flavors of mixed vegetables, frozen is the way to go.

So, these are the main advantages of frozen vegetables. Be sure to stock up on your favorites so you always have some handy, as this will help keep your diet nutritionally sound with very little effort.

Having a Vegetable Garden

There are many families today who have kitchen gardens that they use to produce their own food. If you are interested in more sustainable living, a vegetable garden is a wonderful supplement to a family diet.

Do you find that vegetables from the supermarket these days are tasteless and it seems like, before you know it, they have gone bad? Most of the vegetables that you pick from your garden will be eaten right away. Vegetables from your garden will contain more nutrients than those vegetables that you buy from the store. These vegetables are picked green, and then over their several days journeys to your local market, they ripen.

A garden usually has a compost pile and a few plots of land that are intended to grow one or more kinds of plant in each plot. One of the first things you need to think about is what kind of vegetables would you like to grow? A little planning will help to ensure that you have a productive and enjoyable garden. Try and position your vegetable garden close to your kitchen, so that you have quick and easy access to your harvest.

One vital requirement for a successful vegetable garden is that it is placed in a sunny location. A good vegetable garden must have six hours of full sun every day for your crops to mature properly. Having your rows running north to south will ensure the best sun exposure for your vegetable garden. Healthy soil is another important requirement for a productive vegetable garden. When using fertilizer, make sure it does not contain any herbicides and stay away from pine bark mulches as they are not a good choice for your garden.

There are several ways that you can make the most of your garden space. You can create a raised bed by simply mounding up the soil or you can surround soil in a wood frame, stones, or even concrete. Place the tallest crops like peas, beans, and corn, on the north side of the vegetable garden. The center of the vegetable garden is for the medium-sized crops like cauliflower, broccoli, or tomatoes. Having a vegetable garden can be an enjoyable pastime that will add color, smell, and life to your yard.

People who have large gardens and yards or, people who garden yearly, will find that having a tractor for light work and cultivation, is a good investment. If there is heavy work, like plowing a field, a big tractor is a great investment. You have a wide variety of garden tools to choose from when it comes to working in your garden. Sharp, clean, high-grade tools make your gardening work easier. When it comes to fertilizing your garden, you could do it by hand if your garden is small, or with a wheel type of distributor if you have a large garden.

List of Vegetables

Today, everyone is aware that vegetables are good for you and eating the right amount can improve longevity significantly.

Many people are conscious of the fact that eating five or more portions of different fruits and vegetables a day encourages good health and reduces the risk of chronic diseases such as cancer, heart disease, and diabetes.

VEGETABLES THAT CONTAIN VITAMIN A

Vitamin A is essential for healthy eyes, skin and a strong immune system.

The Vitamin A found in colorful vegetables, usually bright yellow, orange or green is called Provitamin which is then turned into vitamin A within the body.

Here is a list of vegetables that contain vitamin A:

- Asparagus
- Potatoes
- Pumpkin
- Carrots
- Peas
- Broccoli
- Cabbage

It is unlikely you would need to take a supplement to top up your levels of vitamin A if you have a healthy balanced diet. However, if you do feel the need to take vitamin tablets it is always best to seek medical advice before doing so.

VEGETABLES THAT CONTAIN VITAMIN C

Vitamin C is vital to maintain a healthy immune system, large doses can also reduce the chances of catching a cold, help reduce damage to inflamed joints in arthritis sufferers and even reduce many symptoms that asthmatics experience.

Good sources of vegetables with vitamin C are:

- Cabbage
- Spinach
- Peppers
- Broccoli
- Brussels Sprouts
- Cauliflower
- Onions
- Lettuce
- Asparagus
- Cucumber

These vegetables are not only very easy to prepare and cook but are readily available to purchase in supermarkets and farm stores.

VEGETABLES CONTAINING VITAMIN E

Vitamin E is an important antioxidant; it helps to repair cells and is often found in anti-aging creams.

Recent research has shown that this vitamin can delay or even prevent cancer, heart disease and cataracts. The list of vegetables below may be small but very beneficial.

- Spinach
- Broccoli
- Greens

Most vegetables that contain this vitamin are green and leafy. To get the maximum benefit from the above list of vegetables it is recommended you buy organically produced and eat them when they are fresh.

It is a common misconception that eating raw vegetables is better than cooking them. This is not always the case and it really depends on what you want to get out of them. For example, cooking vegetables such as carrots can release certain substances that help us to absorb the vitamins easily.

VEGETABLES THAT HELP REVERSE DIABETES

Vegetables are good for diabetics. Vegetables help diabetics in winning the battle against diabetes. There are many kinds of vegetarian diets. The vegetarian diet is a mix of fruits, vegetables, lentils, grains, nuts and seeds. Vegetables are generally low in calories, fats, and cholesterol. Several health advantages are offered to diabetics by lowering the intake of animal products. Diabetics who choose a vegetarian diet are at lesser risk of high blood pressure, cardiovascular problems, and obesity.

Generally, all vegetables are healthier for diabetics and greatly affect diabetes symptoms; however, there are some vegetables that help to heal the pancreatic function. These vegetables help in controlling the level of blood glucose. A short list of vegetables that help diabetics in diabetes cure sis given below.

Bitter Gourd

This is a folk medicine for diabetics. It is rich in ores, essential vitamins, and iron. It is specifically good for those diabetics who are undernourished. It helps to increase body resistance against different infections.

Bengal Gram

The experiments have proven that water extract of Bengal gram helps in utilizing the glucose. Drinking ½ cup juice of bitter gourd and germinated black germ with a spoonful of honey is a beneficial treatment of a mild type of diabetes.

Groundnut

Daily consumption of groundnut will help the diabetics by checking the development of any vascular complication. It also prevents malnutrition in diabetic patients.

So next time you plan your meals for the week it is better to incorporate these vegetables. The above-mentioned list of vegetables will not only improve the glucose levels but at the same time, it is equally good for the overall general health of the person.

Cautions for Antioxidant Vegetables

With the right antioxidant vegetables, however, you can eat as many as you want how many times you want it and not gain a pound. Employ caution, however, by deciding on the proper kinds of vegetables, because not all of them will maintain your proper weight. "How can that be?" you ask. Well, believe it or not, there are certain vegetables that are excessive in calories while there are, in addition, those that are low in calories. So which vegetables are considered low calorie?

The following are the varieties of antioxidant vegetables that are believed to have low calories and are good to eat if you're in a diet or yearn to lose weight. The list includes carrots, cucumbers, radishes, fresh green beans, celery, cauliflower, cabbage, cherry tomatoes, mushrooms, and lettuce. Obviously, it's unnecessary for you to eat all green vegetables if you are using a vegetable diet. If you look at the choices, you can make your own determination that these not only contain the least calories, they are filled with essential nutrients and antioxidants as well.

To be more precise, should you be in the midst of a low-carbohydrate diet you may have been hearing that munching on vegetables is the path to take. However, just as there are vegetables that include low and high calories, there are also vegetables that are low and high in carbohydrates. Do not generalize that since some antioxidants are in vegetables, they are instantly low in carbohydrates. Vegetables that are low in carbohydrates comprise, but are not limited to, sprouts, leafy greens, hearty greens, herbs, sea vegetables, broccoli, mushrooms, avocado, peppers, summer squash, scallions, asparagus, bamboo shoots, leeks, eggplants, artichoke hearts, okra and more. Of course, veggies with low calories also are short in carbohydrates so you can take your choice.

You might want to use some caution with some high carb vegetables so, here's a listing of vegetables that are starchy and are soaring in carbohydrates. These include beets, corn, parsnips, peas, all types of potatoes, as well as winter squashes. If you wish to experiment on different sorts of vegetables, as there are many to be had in the produce section, you can examine their calorie and carbohydrate count on the internet to lead you on your diet.

Other kinds of vegetables that should be included in your antioxidant diet list are those full of fiber. Don't be perplexed by this declaration. Though vegetables, in general, are good sources of fiber. There are certain forms of vegetables that include more fiber than others. Some great examples of vegetables that are rich in fiber include brussels sprouts, carrots, cooked beans and peas, and spinach. Cruciferous vegetables are also good sources of fiber such as fennel, artichoke, and rutabagas. These vegetables are superior sources of soluble fiber. Soluble fiber will make your stomach have the sensation that it is full and for that reason makes it easier for you to avoid consuming excessive food.

While vegetables are generally not harmful if you are on a diet, observing the correct serving sizes will help speed up the results you want to see. The National Cancer Institute has recommended certain serving sizes for various types of vegetables. The suggested serving size if you are eating uncooked non-leafy vegetables or cooked vegetables is half a cup. If you are consuming raw leafy vegetables, the recommended serving size is one cup. If cooked peas or beans are what you're eating for your meal, the recommended serving size you might take is half a cup.

These serving size recommendations are considered nourishing and aid in dieting as well. Since all the vegetables mentioned previously don't all include the same quantity of carbohydrates, it is still helpful to complete a carbohydrate count on those you want to be included in your diet. A good detail to keep in mind at the time you are calculating your carbohydrates is to eliminate the fiber count as this is normally not included. The reason being there are two types of fiber: insoluble and soluble. The insoluble fiber is about two-thirds of what you eat, it creates bulkier stool, provides no calories and has no effect on blood insulin levels.[1] While the other third is soluble, it dissolves in water. Because so, it slows down foods movement through your body which help make you feel full. [2] After arriving in your colon, soluble fibers are fermented into short chain fatty acids (SCFAs) by bacteria. These SCFAs help keep your gut healthy and may also provide a number of other health benefits. Studies have shown that the fermentation of 1 gram of soluble fiber to SCFA provides about

1–2 calories, depending on the type of fiber (3,4). Since about one-third of the fiber in most foods is soluble, a serving of food containing 6 grams of fiber would contribute up to 4 calories in the form of SCFAs.5

While you are on an antioxidant vegetable diet, keeping a few tips in mind to be careful is crucial. Maybe you lost weight, but you got sick in the process so what's good in that? When you choose vegetables, make an effort to go to the organic produce area. If you find it impossible to acquire organically grown items then apply caution by washing your vegetables thoroughly. Vegetables that are not organically grown include pesticides that are damaging to your well-being.

When you are choosing vegetables, go for the freshest options. You can distinguish when a vegetable is fresh because it is brightly colored and is damage-free or has the slightest amount of blemishes. In-season vegetables are sure to be newly picked so acquiring vegetables growing in their season is a good initiative. You shouldn't plan the continuing storage of vegetables for too long. Buy only the vegetables you plan to be eating in a few days. Other than that, you may get rid of any vegetables that you may have stored too long. When you eat vegetables, aim to leave as much edible skin on them as possible. The skin on vegetables includes their own antioxidant containing substances that can advance your health.

Eating vegetables unprocessed is also a good idea as cooking them can take away some of the nutrients and add fat from the oil you used.

As you can see, antioxidant vegetables may appear intimidating aren't in the least. These are great, fast and low-cost alternatives to fatty foods that bring on the ounces on your weighing scale. As they are minimal in fat, cholesterol, sodium, and calories naturally, it is no wonder that vegetables have been advocated dieters for such a long time. If the recipe is your dilemma, there are great recipe books or online recipes that show you great methods to make your vegetables scrumptious without adding needless fat and eliminating their nutrients.

Fruits

There is an almost universal confusion between a fruit and a vegetable. Some products from trees qualify as vegetables, while others are difficult to classify. Many people believe that vegetables are supposed to be cooked before eating, while their counterparts are eaten raw. Here is where the debate begins because there are those vegetables that do not require to be cooked before consumption. Do they qualify as fruits then?

If we look at the botanical definitions, we find that fruit is defined as the ripened reproductive body of a seed plant. The reproductive body is the ovary and this, therefore, translates to mean that the ripened ovary is the fruit. The ovary ripens after fertilization with a male seed. Many of the ripened ovaries contain seeds in them and the seeds, when planted, are what give rise to a tree or plant that bears the ovaries.

These fruit products are recognized by their ability to produce seeds. However, not all of them contain seeds and some are actually known to be false. For example, the fig tree produces some products that look like they are edible, sweet but are not in real sense. Most of those used in cooking have simply been given the name culinary fruits.

Importance of Fruit

Why eat fruit for optimal diet health? The fruit is loaded with things that are healthy for your body, like antioxidants. Antioxidants are substances that help your body fight free radicals (toxins) that are found in your environment in the form of pollution and in your food as chemicals and preservatives.

Free radicals can do immense harm to your body. They are the reason that now more than any other time in history more people are sick with a disease, more people are on prescription medications, and more people are obese. Even children as young as five and six are being diagnosed with diabetes.

However, if you go to parts of the world where people don't have access to a diet of processed, chemical-laden food you won't find much illness, obesity, or ill health at all. As a matter of fact, the average life span and level of the overall health of individuals in these areas is significantly higher than that of people in the United States or Europe.

Why is the general health of individuals in these areas better? It is because their diet health revolves around a lot of organic fruit. Organic whole foods don't contain any free radicals because they are grown naturally without any:

- Pesticides
- Artificial fertilizers
- Growth hormones
- Preservatives
- Chemicals

The antioxidants that are in fruit (the highest concentrations are in dark-colored fruits) fight free radicals and slow down the aging process. The Acai berry, from the Amazon rainforest, has enough antioxidants to help fight diseases like cancer. The goji and noni berry have been found to have similar diet health benefits.

FRUIT FOR YOUR BRAIN'S HEALTH

Believe it or not, adding fruit to your diet can give you a more efficient memory. This is because when you eat "living" foods, such as fruit, they are perfect nutrition for your "living" cells, which make up your brain and every other part of your body. If your cells are thriving and healthy, that corresponding part of the body will have improved function as well.

FIBER

For optimal diet health, you need fiber. Fiber ensures a healthy digestive system, which is responsible for the final task in eliminating free radicals from your body. Consuming adequate fiber is also key in fighting and reducing the risk of getting diseases like colon cancer.

Making organic fruit a part of your diet and health helps your body fight and prevent many unwanted things such as:

- Heart disease
- Obesity
- Diabetes
- Alzheimer's
- Cataracts
- Stroke

As you can see there are many reasons to reach for a piece of fruit rather than a candy bar or bag of potato chips when you want a snack. Of course, you can indulge in whatever you want occasionally. However, if you can eat more fruit you will notice the diet health benefits fairly quick.

Vegetables and Fruits That Improve Sexual Health

There are many foods that can contain nutrients that are required for good sexual health. In order to have good stimulating arousal, our body needs a mixture of vitamins and trace elements. Plants are the category of foods that offer the most abundance, and people often regard vegetables and fruits as the best sources of nutrients.

Back in ancient times, humanity has been infatuated with aphrodisiacs for many years. It's been found that some aphrodisiacs are not as pleasurable as they once were, sadly some proven dangerous. Fortunately, there is a safe and sure way to boost your love libido without dampening desire and sensuality. Nature gives us a vast variety of colorful delicious plants. Some of these plants provide specific functions for both men and women, for instance:

THE VALUE OF POMEGRANATE

Whether you eat or drinkpomegranate, this plant provides great benefits. Pomegranate is a plant that is able to enhance erections and reduce erectile dysfunction. There are scientific studies showing a promoted blood flow to the penis, with the use of rabbits in experiments. This research, published in the Journal of Urology, shows the possibility of a cure for erectile dysfunction. This process is a very complex matter and according to Wikipedia, the mechanism underneath is still not very clear, but scientists are confident that increasing zinc, trace elements, vitamin A, B1, B3 and vitamin C, and omega three fatty acids nutrient levels in the body can improve and help stimulate conditions.

EAT MORE SPINACH

If you never liked spinach before, maybe this will change your mind. This small green leafy vegetable is amazing, it is rich in magnesium. Magnesium is a mineral that lessens inflammation in blood vessels, increasing blood flow. According to sex expert Dr. Tammy Nelson, " increased blood flow sends blood to your lower extremities, which, escalate arousal and allows you to have sex more pleasurable," women will find it is easier to have an orgasm.

Nuts

Omega 3 fatty acids are known to be good for reducing cholesterol levels. This is because the fatty acids are able to relax arteries and blood vessels, so that blood can flow smoothly within our body causing stimulation for women and men.

Citrus Fruits

Citrus fruits are rich in vitamin C, an important nutrient for our body. It is also beneficial to the condition of sperm, as it can keep sperm from clumping together. Vitamin C provides sperm with a better foundation to find the ovum, so that sperm motility, an important factor for fertilization, can be improved.

Bananas

Banana is a very good fruit for humans. It raises our body condition in all aspects because it is rich in nutrients. It contains not only vitamins but also many amino acids which are good for mental health. Not to mention the trace elements like magnesium and potassium. While you should already know the importance of magnesium (discussed in spinach),

Figs

Figs are rich in amino acids. Amino acids are the raw materials for hormones including testosterone, the sexual hormone. Therefore, deficiency of amino acids not only gives you poor body health but also weaker erection, lower sex drive and libido for women and men.

Onions

Onion has a nutrient called allicin. This allicin is phytochemical in nature, and it can thin the blood so that blood circulation is improved.

Celery

Celery is able to promote testosterone production so that your sexual stamina can be improved.

Cherries and berries

Cherries and berries are rich in anthocyanins, which can prevent cholesterol from blocking the arteries and capillaries.

Chilis

Chilis increase our rate of blood circulation and expand our blood vessels. More blood is pumped into capillaries (including penile blood vessels).

CHAPTER EIGHT

Laughter: Good For Your Health

This is something I love to do and I am able to feel immediate affects from doing so. Laughter. Did you know that when you respond to the everyday stresses of life with an overabundance of Negative Emotional Responses (NER) such as anxiety, anger, or hostility you are significantly increasing your risk of developing heart disease, and many others? What do all of these negative emotions have in common; can you guess what emotion underlies them all? The underlying emotion that drives us to feel anxiety, anger, and hostility is fear.

The question I am going to propose to you is this, what scares you so much about living a life that you are afraid to live it up to its full capacity? How much do you, happily, laugh at yourself and with others? How often you laugh at life, can definitely provide some positive, physical health effects.

In fact, an official research study undertaken by cardiologists at the University of Maryland Medical Center in Baltimore, back in November 2000, headed by Dr. Michael Miller, M.D., revealed for the first time just how healthy it really is to laugh.

This investigation originally consisted of 300 participants. Half (150) of the test subjects were healthy and age-matched with another 150 test subjects, who had suffered a heart attack or who had undergone coronary artery bypass surgery. A subsequent study that has been conducted since the first one, by the way, confirms earlier findings, in that laughter seems to increase blood flow to the 'endothelium,' the tissue that forms the inner lining of blood vessels.

Fearful emotions were shown to restrict blood flow, while the opposite was true during episodes of extreme happiness. Overall, average blood flow increased by 22 percent during and after bouts of laughter, while blood flow decreased by 35 percent during mental stress. It is also worth mentioning here, that the positive health effects of laughing were experienced for up to several hours after the joyful event. The same can be said for a stressful event. So, being mindful of what life events you let upset you would be wise.

Miller's study indicated that heart disease patients who took life or themselves too seriously were 40 percent less likely to laugh at a wide variety of common, everyday life situations when compared to their healthy age-related counterparts.

Laughing it up can, and does, help counteract the negative effects of chronic stress on the body. Besides increasing blood flow in blood vessels, surprising results also show that laughing appears to increase your immune system response, lowers blood sugar levels in diabetics, and helps induce a state of relaxation promoting better sleep.

More good news, when you are laughing it up you are increasing the oxygen flow throughout your entire body system, benefiting at both the cellular and organ level. Repetition at gasping for air over something uncontrollably funny is akin to a short-term hyperventilation session. Ever heard of an oxygen bar? If you have, try to have a good laugh while you are there, too. Because, when you are taking in huge amounts of air while you are laughing, just like you are partaking of at an oxygen bar, it increases your energy on an intracellular level that is important to sustaining human life.

A good hearty laugh, while it boosts the circulation of your blood and oxygen flow, will also give you quite an abdominal work-out. Looking for a fun way to achieve those six-pack abs you admire so much? What better way can you think of to help you get those stomach muscles in shape? It will also help exercise facial muscles. Ever laughed so hard that your sides ached and your face was tired? Problem is, we don't get nearly enough of these kinds of laughs as we ought to.

The biochemical release related to this type of amusement is not, scientifically, well understood. However, what is understood is that brain chemical releases such as serotonin (among many others) and immune system chemicals called 'interleukins' are known to be involved. Imagine what the major pharmaceutical companies would charge us for these types of naturally released chemical compounds if they could synthesize and bottle them.

All you have to do to get these though is to freely improve your greater outlook on life in general. So, how can you possibly do this? A few ideas come to mind.

1. Try to spend more time around friends or family with a good sense of humor, and who make you feel good.

2. Watch a group of children interact with each other while playing.

3. Rent some funny movies, or watch a live comedy improv show, or on television.

4. Imagine some of your stuffier co-workers without clothing on. How funny would they look if they weren't hiding behind their fashion label apparel?

The bottom line is this, to benefit from the health effects of laughing, emotionally and physically, you must actively try to look for more humor in everyday life situations. Take note when a certain situation is making you feel uptight, threatened, or fearful. Remember, fear is only useful and necessary when it involves saving your life; it's not for experiencing on a daily basis.

The future recommendations for reducing chronic stress that may result in heart disease, or any other life-altering health condition, just might be to properly exercise routinely, eat and drink wisely, and get in a few good bellies laughs as often as you can. In doing this, we would all become a little bit healthier, and certainly, feel happier with our world.

Physiological Benefits of Laughter

Many studies have looked at the benefits laughter brings to the body. When we laugh, it triggers the part of the brain known as the nucleus acumens, which in turn releases the chemical dopamine. When dopamine is released, the mood is increased. Furthermore, laughter helps release muscle tension in our bodies helping us to relax. It affects the diaphragm, abdominal muscles and shoulders.

Laughter is good for the heart, which is also a muscle. The research found that watching a funny movie improves blood-vessel function. Such a change helps reduce the risk of cardiovascular disease. It can also help lower blood pressure. In addition, it can bring a boost to the immune system, therefore helping to keep illness at bay. When we laugh there is increased production of immune cells and gamma interferon which serve to raise immunity.

In 1979 Norman Cousins prescribed his own laughter therapy which involved watching episodes of the Marx Brothers and Candid Camera. He suffered from ankylosing spondylitis (which inflames the joints and the spine) and found the therapy not only reduced his pain but also decreased inflammation. According to Cousins, laughter releases endorphins, which help relieve pain. Presumably, then it can aid people who suffer from chronic pain.

Some research has suggested that laughing burns more calories. Laughing out loud at a comedy was shown to burn 20% more calories and increased heart rate compared to watching a run of the mill documentary.

Laughter can be a great antidote to stress. When we are stressed, the hormone cortisol enters the bloodstream. If left unmanaged (i.e. you remain in a stressed state), it can cause problems, including high blood pressure, lowered immunity and blood sugar imbalance, which can lead to diabetes. However, laughter has been found to lower cortisol levels.

Psychological Benefits of Laughter

As we have seen, laughter is a great way to reduce the physical symptoms of stress. It also helps us out psychologically and is a great way to relieve tension. Being able to laugh at life, yourself and your situation puts you in a better position for coping. It can even help prevent burnout for people in highly demanding jobs, such as health care professionals working with terminally ill patients.

Having laughter in your life can act as a buffer against the reality that life isn't always great. The research found humor was associated with a return to life satisfaction for those who had suffered physical illness. It may also aid recovery from depression. Recent research at the University of Utah found that recently bereaved spouses who experienced more humor and laughter in their lives had a better adjustment to their loss, suffering less grief and depression as a result.

Being able to laugh at yourself and the mistakes you make helps you recognize that when mistakes happen they are not the end of the world. Seeing the lighter side of life really helps put things into perspective. Life cannot be all bad if there is still something to laugh about. It can help a person rise to a challenge, rather than be defeated by it. Not surprising then, it is an indication of good self-esteem. You are able to put your guard down and allow people to see that you are open to having fun. Also, you are not worrying about what other people think.

Overall, laughter offers a person greater wellbeing and a sense of control. It can help a person recognize that life and its difficulties aren't being forced on them.

Social Benefits of Laughter

Laughter is a social thing. Although you can sit and watch a funny film on your own, it is always a pleasure to laugh with friends and share jokes and funny stories. The great thing about laughter is it is contagious. You laugh, others laugh. So many people can benefit from what started out as one person's chuckle. Not surprisingly, laughter can help lessen con-flicts—providing people are laughing together rather than at the expense of another.

Laughter can help bring people together. Research by Fraley and Aron supports this idea. Pairs of strangers worked together either on a task that brought about laughter or on a more serious task. Afterward, the strangers who had laughed together liked their partner more and felt closer to them.

Humor also plays an important role in the workplace. It can bring enjoyment and increase feelings of cohesion. It can bring colleagues closer as they laugh about issues that only those who work there would understand. Importantly, it can help release tensions that have been building within the work environment for some time.

Tips for Injecting Regular Laughter into Your Life

You shouldn't really need these tips, as everybody knows how to laugh. Yet sometimes life can get a bit much, so it's always good to be aware of laughter opportunities.

- Laugh at yourself. This may not be easy, but life doesn't seem nearly as bad when you are able to do this. You don't have to be disparaging, just when you mess up, say something silly and so on. You will feel more confident when you don't take yourself or life so seriously. Let your defenses down for a moment and laugh instead.

- Go see a comedian.

- Don't be afraid to laugh out loud in public. Don't stifle your laugh. Worried people will stare at you? Who cares—think of the benefits that laugh offers. Remember laughter is contagious.

- Laugh with others rather than at others. It is important to make this distinction. (Making a fool of another in order to get a laugh is not the way forward.)

- Look for the lighter side of a situation. Even if you don't share it with others, be aware it is there.

- Make someone laugh. Make an effort to cheer up a friend or family member. Look for opportunities to bring a smile to a child's face.

- Try some laughter yoga. This is a relatively new concept that combines the benefits of laughter with the benefits of yoga. Classes are available in 60 countries.

- Read websites that make you laugh.

- Read light-hearted books.

- Watch your favorite comedy.

- Share funny memories with your friends and family.

- When you have a bad start to the day, laugh about it with others. Don't let it ruin the rest of your day.

- The next time you are at home ill, stick a comedy on. It'll help pass the time, raise your spirits and you may get better sooner.

- Don't be a grouchy boss. Employees appreciate the humor in their managers and work more effectively as a consequence.

Humor is a personal thing. As such, you can be the one who decides what comedies are funny and which comedians make you laugh. Don't waste your time watching something that only irritates you, believing you should find it funny.

As you go about your day, keep a lookout for fun things to make you

Stop Drinking Alcohol

and other people laugh. It can change how you perceive the world.

What is alcoholism really? Here is some information that will dispel some of the myths about how alcoholism works, and how it will affect your life. Your normal drinker can enjoy a mixed drink or a glass of wine, or even two or three. A person who has become an alcoholic generally can't stop drinking once they get started, drink heavy volume, and it will affect their life in a somewhat predictable way if the drinking continues.

The Myths about Alcoholism

There is information everywhere written by people not genuinely qualified to define or describe alcoholism. If they haven't experienced it themselves, they are just collecting information, guessing for the most part of what alcoholism really is and what it entails, from a strictly "outside" point of view.

And the truth of the matter is alcohol isn't just a physical addiction that can be driven out of your body in 72 hours (which is standard thinking on the subject) which in itself is a myth—closer to a year would be the truth, and further is also an incredibly powerful emotional addiction. This emotional addiction routinely reaches the point where you cannot picture your life without alcohol.

Alcohol Abuse

There are some descriptions of alcohol abuse where it is defined as a person who drinks regularly, but who also maintains their responsibilities, while at the same time occasionally putting themselves in jeopardy for example by driving under the influence, and sometimes drinking large quantities. Anyone who drinks every day, even if it is controlled drinking, is most likely an alcoholic unless it is, for instance, a drink before dinner.

There are alcoholics who are highly functional with controlled drinking for decades, making it work every day, possibly holding a highly responsible job for instance. Conventional thinking on this is if you drink every day, you still may not be physically dependent on it. First, if you are drinking every day, it is doubtful that you are not physically addicted, but more importantly, this concept completely ignores the tremendous emotional addiction aspect of drinking. And some of these daily drinkers will tell you the job was the last thing to go. Drinking daily may put you in the alcoholic category.

BINGE DRINKING

The habit of occasionally drinking very large quantities of alcohol is considered binge drinking. Contrary to popular belief, binge drinking can be an ongoing occurrence throughout a person's entire life. It is not limited to high school or college years. Binge drinking has no age limit. And after a person has been binge drinking for years and years, starting when they were young in most cases, they could also be considered an alcoholic.

THE NEED TO DRINK

Alcoholism has gray areas, but when you reach that point where drinking is affecting your life in an adverse way, you are going to know you have a problem. One major sign is you have an overwhelming need to drink. There is no way to win when you are up against alcohol no matter how strong or disciplined you are. The best possible alcoholic scenario is if you are a highly functioning alcoholic and can pull it off for decades. However, alcohol still takes its toll here, as it does in every single case with no exception. As a highly functional drinker, when you drink every day, the alcohol will affect your health (your vital organs) and will cause liver and brain damage.

So, what "experts" who don't have a drinking problem don't understand (among other things) is once alcohol gets you it takes over your life—physically and emotionally. You have a need to drink, and the longer you drink, the greater the need. You learn to rely on alcohol, and in the beginning, it doesn't disappoint, but as the problem grows alcohol turns on you, and becomes a very personal, formidable enemy.

Effects of Alcohol

Alcohol comes in to disrupt the natural metabolism system and functions of the brain very quickly after the drink is consumed. Before it reaches the brain, alcohol is absorbed through blood vessels located in the wall of the stomach and small intestine. Within minutes only, alcohol travels from the stomach to the brain and affects the nerves. From the total amounts of alcohol consumed, as much as 20% is processed in the stomach and the rest of it is absorbed via the small intestine.

As we all have been informed, the liver should metabolize alcohol and eliminate the toxic substances from the blood. Nevertheless, the liver can only process some amount of alcohol one at a time; the un-processed liquor will be freely circulating in the bloodstream. Its effects on the body depend greatly on the amount of the un-metabolized liquor consumed. Overconsumption of alcohol can also disrupt the respiratory system. In some cases, blood cannot absorb oxygen, thus the brain does not function at all. It can cause coma or death.

Long term effects of alcohol are very dangerous such as brain impairment and permanent liver malfunction. Added to a poor diet, alcohol can affect the entire health condition. Most likely, visible symptoms are emotional difficulties in the form of depression and bad relationships. Possibly, long terms effects of alcohol are likely to be:

- Loss of memory, hallucination, brain injury, confusion

- Loss of muscle tissue and weakness

- Cancer of liver, mouth, and throat

- Irregular heartbeats, high blood pressure

- Stomach ulcers, inflamed stomach lining

- Inflamed pancreas

- Damaged sperm, shrinking of testicles, impotence

- Gynecological problems

Provided that everybody has a different metabolism system in terms of speed and daily diets, alcohol does what it does in different manners as well. Blood Alcohol Concentration (BAC) is the most helpful guide to decide what alcohol can do to a certain drinker.

Anyway, liquor does not need to wait for long before any kind of effect is produced in the body. Within only five minutes, alcohol starts to produce chemical reactions in the brain. One standard amount of alcohol will lead BAC to be in its highest state after 30 to 45 minutes. When multiple amounts are consumed within the time, BAC will only get higher faster than expected by the blood and body. The human metabolism system can completely break down one standard amount of liquor in one hour. The final results or effects of alcohol on the body depend greatly on:

- Health condition

- Quantity of alcohol consumed

- Type of liquor

- Body chemistry

- Diets

- Age

- Drinking experience

- Mental/psychological condition and more.

To avoid either short or long-term effects of alcohol, simply follow the guidelines provided by the National Health and Medical Research Council. The guidelines help to reduce the percentage of risk factors both short and long terms effects. The followings are some of the most essential rules included in the guidelines:

- On any day, either men or women cannot drink more than one standard amount of alcohol to reduce the risk factor of alcohol-related diseases or permanent damage in the body as the result of long-term effects of alcohol.

- On any one occasion, either men or women should never take more than four standard amounts of alcohol to reduce the chance of having alcohol-related-injury as short term effects.

SOCIAL EFFECTS OF ALCOHOL

If you are having trouble with alcoholism, it is not only you who is affected but also the family. They will be the ones to take care of you when you get drunk, pay for the damages that you did while you were drunk and be there to support until you overcome the problem. Because of this, they will have less time for themselves, to study or work and do other things that they want to do because of you. Also, alcohol addiction can lead to increased tension, quarreling, depression, behavior problems and work problems resulting in relationships becoming unstable which eventually leads to domestic violence and divorce.

Outside the family, alcoholism can bring damages to society. There can be higher rates of crimes such as fraud, sexual offenses, libel, theft, driving offenses and other criminal charges that could be done especially when an alcoholic is out of his mind while doing things. Aside from these, accidents are very much prevalent. Many people drink and drive and get injured or die. It also happens that there are others who get injured or die in accidents. Before the worst unexpected scenario comes, be a responsible person, family member and member of the society and drink alcohol moderately.

MENTAL AND PSYCHOLOGICAL EFFECTS OF ALCOHOL

The effects that alcoholism has on the body are well-documented. Everyone knows how excessive alcohol intake can lead to rapid deterioration of personal health and internal organs. What is discussed less frequently, but in many ways equally damaging, is the toll alcohol abuse takes on the mind. The following are some of the most significant mental effects of alcoholism and how they negatively impact the individual.

DIMINISHED SELF-ESTEEM

The behavior of the alcoholic leads them to be looked down upon by family and friends. This often leads to lower self-esteem, which can perpetuate the cycle of problem drinking. Simply put, the worse a person feels about themselves, the more likely they are to go looking for escape in a bottle. This loss of self-esteem can lead to other problems as well, including poor performance at work and withdrawal in common social situations.

POOR JUDGMENT

The alcoholic makes bad decisions. During their impaired state under the influence, they are likely to lie to the people they care about, steal, or engage in other destructive mental behavior. The alcoholic becomes a person that nobody wants to be around.

REDUCED INHIBITIONS

Problem drinking causes many people to temporarily lose their inhibitions. This can lead to a multitude of problems—all associated with unprotected sex with multiple partners. These serious issues include sexually transmitted diseases, unwanted or unplanned pregnancy, and rape.

LOSS OF SEXUAL INTEREST

Alternatively, individuals can experience "coin," which is reduced inhibitions. This is the lack of sexual interest brought on by alcoholism. Many alcoholics replace the love and affection of their partners with the solace they find in their drinking. Also, erectile dysfunction becomes more prevalent in heavy drinkers—leading to abstinent behavior with the alcoholic's spouse or significant other.

EXAGGERATED EMOTIONS

Alcoholics are prone to extreme moods and mood swings. Unable to cope with problems on a national level, the alcoholic will grow deeply depressed at the smallest things and have a hard time bouncing back from the curve balls life throws at us all. Conversely, the problem drinker may get extremely happy and excitable during a drinking binge, only to "crash and burn" when that high period ends.

MEMORY LOSS

An alcoholic is likely to drink so much that they experience blackouts—periods where they cannot remember anything about their actions. Memory loss due to alcohol abuse is psychologically damaging and highly self-destructive in nature. Although he personally has no memory of it, the alcoholic may say or do things to friends and family, that leave emotional scars that take a great deal of time to heal.

INCREASED AGGRESSION

Violent, aggressive behavior is common among male (and many times female) alcoholics. The loss of inhibitions, coupled with the destruction of brain cells caused by drinking can create abusive behavior in alcohol abusers. Spousal abuse and street fighting are often the result of alcoholism and binge drinking.

Effects of Alcohol Abuse on Children

Alcohol abuse doesn't only affect the drinker. Children can be negatively impacted as well. With a parent who is experiencing significant mental issues associated with alcoholism, the child's development may be stunted—they have a good chance of growing up with significant learning and anger management issues. Without a reliable parent, the child is liable to grow up lacking the trust and self-confidence necessary to succeed.

It's obvious that alcoholism affects behavior as much as it does our physical capacities. The psychological impact of alcoholism, however, is in many ways worse than the physical counterpart, because it not only affects the drinker himself but those around him as well.

Ways to Stop Drinking Alcohol

You may be one of those who want to know how to stop drinking alcohol on your own. There are a lot of reasons for an individual to decide to stop drinking alcohol. It might be that you easily get drunk. You have admitted to yourself that you are an alcoholic. Or you have admitted that it isn't healthy at all. Whatever your reason is, it is up to the individual for the success of this decision.

First and foremost, you must have a strong will to stop drinking alcohol. You have made the decision on your own, determined to be successful. According to some researchers, once you have decided you must have an inspiration to stay committed on your decision. This would be a big help for you. Family and friends are the biggest support one could have.

Once you know you have your family and friends' support you must stay away from temptation. If there are empty bottles around your house, dispose of them. You, yourself know how strong or weak you are when tempted to stop drinking alcohol on your own. There should be no temptation at your home.

Though you can't avoid it if you're in a party, be determined to say "no." If you're on a slow withdrawal process, drink just a small amount. Or if you can bring someone with you at the party much better, your friend or companion could watch over you. It is better if someone is there to remind you of your decision. Inspiration is always a big help.

Let your colleagues know about your decision, so they could also help you. There are instances that drinks are offered at work. When your colleagues know that you are stopping from drinking alcohol they could help you with these instances.

Ending alcohol consumption and behaviors on your own is not an easy road to take. You must go through a lot. Stay away from those who don't support your decision. This means your list of friends will be affected or your social life will be limited. But this would be a part of your success. Bad influences are not good for someone who is starting to quit drinking.

These are just some of the ways on how to stop drinking alcohol on your own. After your admission to stop drinking alcohol you can work out what program you would follow to achieve your goal. The program would depend on an individual's lifestyle and personality. Some would start with a slow reduction of alcohol intake. If you're a frequent drinker, sudden withdrawal will cause mild to severe physical symptoms. Some of these symptoms are:

- Headache

- Shaking

- Sweating

- Nausea or vomiting

- Anxiety and restlessness

- Stomach cramps and diarrhea

- Trouble in sleeping or concentrating

- Elevated heart rate and blood pressure

It is best that you consult a doctor to learn more about the sudden withdrawal that may cause your body.

Alcohol & drug withdrawal can be one of the most difficult things for someone who is dependent on these substances. Yet, if you are a daily user and have a difficult time stopping it may be time for you to think about it and take some action. Alcohol & drug use is a killer in more ways than one. It destroys your body and brain; it can cause depression, weight-gain, violence, as well as other behavior problems; it can destroy relationships and can tear families apart. If you are ready to stop drinking alcohol or using drugs and need some assistance this article will help. I have put together 12 simple & effective steps that can help stop your addiction and change your life! Please read on.

Steps to End Addiction

Here are important steps we can take to stop our addiction:

AVOID STRESS

Stress causes some of us to drink or use drugs. We want to relax and escape. Unfortunately, this does not work as a long-term solution as it causes much more damage than we realize. Avoid stressful situations when withdrawing. Keep calm and centered.

TAKE A BREAK FROM WORK WHEN WITHDRAWING (14–30 DAYS)

Essential! Normal initial "detox" takes about 30 days. The first 14 days are essential for withdrawal. Take a vacation or sick leave or work part-time. Cut down on any triggers that may hurt you. It's your life, protect yourself.

FIND SUPPORT

Find friends, family and/or a comfortable support group. You need to be open with these folks and ask for their support. You need to change friends and settings that do not support your sobriety.

DO A BODY CLEANSE AND DETOX

You need to rid yourself of all those toxins in your body. This will also give you the strength and energy to stay sober. Cleanse for 30 days if possible.

TAKE VITAMINS & SUPPLEMENTS

Your body & brain need help! It is essential to have those extra vitamins and minerals in your body for your recovery.

- **Vitamin C** reduces stress and anxiety.

- **Angelica** is an anti-inflammatory and diaphoretic herb that prevents nausea and ease headache while facing alcohol withdrawal.

- **Basil** eliminates toxins and free radicals from the blood and liver, reduces the alcohol cravings.

- **Acorn** diminishes the craving for alcohol, eases its effect and returns your energy and vitality.

- **Kudzu** is a natural antidote that promotes the regeneration of liver tissues.

EAT HEALTHY FOODS

Healthy eating is another key to recovery. You've got to have the proper nutrition to stay sober and repair your damaged body.

DRINK LIQUIDS

Drink lots of water and herbal tea. Drink 6–8 glasses a day. Avoid high sugar drinks. Hydrate yourself. This helps with cravings and withdrawal. It also helps your body & brain detox and gets healthy.

GET SLEEP

Get regular sleep. This has to do with stress and resting the body & mind. You are recovering from an illness. The more rested you are, the better you will heal.

HAVE A SPIRITUAL/MENTAL PRACTICE

Meditate, pray, reflect, and utilize positive affirmations. Do something to stimulate your belief system. Taking good care of the mind, emotions, and spirit are important for health and recovery.

BREATHE

Focus on the present and get centered by breathing in and out, focusing on nothing else. Air is your life force, concentrate on calming down and focus on relaxing as you take deep breaths for several minutes. Use this technique to reduce stress and gain needed strength.

DON'T GET HUNGRY, ANGRY, LONELY OR TIRED (HALT)

This is an important reminder to be conscious of these powerful triggers. Be aware of these four triggers and take steps to reduce their negative effects.

CHAPTER TEN

Drink Enough Water

RIDE OUT THE CRAVINGS

Craving alcohol or drugs doesn't last forever. It works like a bell curve…it gets really intense then decreases with time. For most people, the intense craving can last about 10–14 days. Remember, it doesn't last forever. Be strong; find support. Utilize the 12 steps above and you will succeed!

It is a fact that the average human needs to consume at least 64 ounces of water every day just to optimize the vital functions within the body. Those who live in hotter climates or who exercise regularly need to take in even more of this precious fluid. Most of us do not consume anywhere near the minimum amount that we need in order to remain healthy.

Our society is geared towards the consumption of soft drinks, coffee, and tea far more than often than we should. Although it seems like we are getting plenty of pure, healthy water when you look at bottled water sales, the truth is that only a fraction of us are contributing to this market. Many people choose flavored drinks because they say that they simply don't like the taste of water.

When it comes to this sort of opposition to drinking enough water facts are that the reason you may not like the taste, smell, or appearance of your water is that it is contaminated. The biggest cause of bad smell and taste is the carcinogenic chlorine that we introduce for purposes of disinfection. The fact is that the thousands of contaminants currently present in our water supply don't even have to affect the appearance or taste of your water in order to affect your health.

Most people that drink water do not realize how many toxins and carcinogens their body is absorbing on a regular basis. This is true even of the bottled water that many of us choose to consume regularly. Bottled water has just as many contaminants in it as tap water does, and just chemicals that leach off the plastic from your bottle alone is enough to eventually cause you to develop cancer.

Since it is vitally important that you are drinking enough water facts about contamination of both tap and bottled water are a major concern. You can avoid having the chemicals, pathogens, and toxic organic compounds present in our water supply affect your life with the purchase and installation of a sophisticated tap water purifying system. Such an appliance will remove up to 99.9% of all contaminant matter present.

Water consumption facts state that you need to do better if you want to improve your health. A home drinking water purification system makes getting enough pure, healthy water easy.

Types of Water for Home Use

Drinking water is now available in different forms. Centuries ago, there was only water from wells. Now, the list goes from distilled to alkaline water. How many types of our precious liquid can companies come up with now? That remains to be seen.

BOTTLED WATER

Most people think that all commercially available bottled water is 100% pure. Well, that is not the case. Some commercially available water is a product of filtration and disinfection. Bottled water is safe to drink because the harmful microorganisms have been killed. There are different ways to kill microorganisms. It could be through the use of chemicals like chlorine or the use of radiation. Traces of minerals may still be present.

DISTILLED WATER

Distillation is one method to purify H_2O. It is a method that is based on the simple principle of the water cycle. Plain H_2O is heated and then the vapor is allowed to condense. Condensed H_2O is collected in another container. The process can be repeated to ensure a high-grade of distillation. The process leaves solid impurities behind. As a result, the remaining distilled liquid is almost devoid of minerals and ions, a quality that according to some people is not good for the body. There has been controversy that distilled water strips the body of minerals. This has been dismissed by some health experts as a myth.

DEIONIZED H_2O

Another way to remove ions from H_2O is deionization. In this process, water is allowed to pass through ion exchange resin beds, where water loses its ions. This process, however, does not remove non-ionic impurities. But when it is done to previously treated H_2O, the result is high-grade pure water.

ALKALINE WATER

This type of processed water has been introduced in the market fairly recently. It is unlike distilled water that is totally devoid of minerals. It may be considered healthier than plain spring water because it contains only the ions necessary for the body. According to promoters of this type of water, it is healthier because it has antioxidants and has healing qualities, claims that have yet to be proven by thorough medical research.

RO WATER

Reverse osmosis is another means of purifying H_2O to some extent. Unlike deionization, it removes all molecules and ions larger than water molecules. Therefore, the result was a purer form of H_2O, much like distilled water.

Importance of Drinking Enough Water

Approximately 75% of our total body weight is made up of water. The majority of the water in our body is found within the intracellular space in the cells. When we have more water leaving our body than we are taking in, dehydration sets in. It only takes 1% or 2% dehydration for our cognitive functioning to start being affected. We lose water through our usual bodily processes such as breathing, sweating, urinating and bowel movements. On any normal day the average person loses approximately 1.5 liters of water through bodily processes, more if they are exercising or it is hotter weather, they have diarrhea or vomiting, or if they are consuming caffeinated drinks such as tea and coffee. Caffeine is a diuretic, meaning it causes the body to lose more water. Therefore, we should all be drinking at least 1.5–2 liters of water to replace what we have lost.

WHAT IF I'M NOT DRINKING ENOUGH WATER?

If it is not replaced and water from within the blood vessels is lost, the body can compensate by shifting water from cells into the blood vessels. However, this is a very short-term solution and symptoms of dehydration will come on quickly if the water is not replaced. By the time the thirst mechanism kicks in the body is quite dehydrated. You can tell whether you are dehydrated by the color of your urine—it should be almost clear or a light straw-color; if you are dehydrated it will be more yellow or dark yellow in color.

As the level of water loss increases, more symptoms of dehydration become apparent such as a dry mouth, the eyes stop making tears, sweating may stop, muscle cramps, nausea and vomiting, heart palpitations and light-headedness (particularly when standing). The body tries to maintain the amount of blood being pumped around the body which may mean the heart rate increases, and this causes blood vessels to constrict to maintain pressure. This may begin to fail as the level of dehydration increases. Water is also very important for removing toxins so if we are dehydrated a build-up of toxins occurs.

With severe dehydration, confusion and weakness will occur as the brain and other body organs receive less blood. If it remains untreated then the worst-case scenario is organ failure and or coma.

Most of us would not get to this level of dehydration. However, time and time again I talk to people who sit at their desks all day long drinking coffee and no water at all because they don't like the taste of it, or because they are not used to making it part of their routine. Coffee is a diuretic meaning it flushes water from the body. I wonder how dehydrated these people are? Being dehydrated also makes you tired—many people when tired at work will just reach for another cup of coffee, which may wake you up for a short while, but the caffeine high quickly results in a tired slump. Did you know that drinking a pint of water is often more effective at waking you up rather than a cup of coffee? And you don't get the caffeine crash afterward.

So, what are the symptoms of dehydration that we in the Western, working world are likely to recognize? About 85% of our brain cells are made up of water, so if the body is lacking in this vital liquid then it is not surprising that the first signs are changes in our cognitive functioning. Being only 2% dehydrated can seriously degrade physical and mental functions, being 15% dehydrated is likely to be lethal.

SYMPTOMS OF MILD TO SEVERE DEHYDRATION:

- Chronic pain in joints and muscles
- Lower back pain

- Headaches

- Constipation

- A strong odor to your urine along with a yellow or amber color

- High thirst

- Rapid weight loss

- Dry mouth and adhesive saliva

- Reduced urination

- Fatigue

- Cold hands and feet

- Increased heart rate

- Loss of appetite

- Changes in behavior such as increased fear, embarrassment and inattention

- Decreased ability of short-term memory and concentration

- Dizziness

SO HOW CAN YOU AVOID DEHYDRATION?

- When you sleep your body doesn't receive any water for several hours. Drink a glass as soon as you wake up—this will also help you to wake up in the morning.

- Drink water slowly throughout the day—don't think that you can get your whole water intake by drinking 1.5 liters in one go, you will feel very sick!

- Keep a bottle of water with you at all times, if sitting at a desk keep it in front of you and keep sipping throughout the day.

- Regularly eat fluid rich fruits and vegetables.

- Avoid salty foods as these can dry you. Don't cut out salt altogether as we do need salt in our diet.

- Limit intake of alcohol and caffeine.

If used to drinking a lot of water it will take some adjusting, especially as you will be going to the loo a lot more! And if you don't like water then try to avoid adding sugary squash, instead try squeezing lemon juice in the glass then filling it with water.

Water is essential to survive. People tend to only drink when they are thirsty, but this is NOT what you should be doing, yet so many people mistake being thirsty for being hungry. You may think that you need food to fill up on, but just drinking a single glass of water can dramatically help you and let you be optimized in your performance.

Lack of water is the prominent cause of constipation, as well as can cause false signs of memory loss and even make you have some heart attack symptoms if not taken care of immediately.

Water cleanses your body and is the only way to flush your body clear of any toxins or waste that is built up. Supplying additional water to yourself daily will drastically help in your digestion and will help you feel freer to do what you want to do, instead of feeling lazy.

You may face a few different signs of being thirsty without even recognizing that you are. If your mouth gets dry, drink some water. If you start to feel hungry, drink some water. If you're going out for a run, take a bottle of water with you so you don't get dehydrated along the way.

Even if your body only drops 2% in water, it could cause problems with your memory or math skills, or very well hinder your efforts to concentrate on simple tasks such as working on the computer. Drinking a decent supply of water (8–10 glasses is HIGHLY recommended), can reduce diseases and cancers dramatically, up to 45% when it comes to colon cancer, and a whopping 79% when it comes to breast cancer.

Not drinking enough water can make you slowly grow blood clots and potentially cause a stroke. But if you supply yourself with enough water you won't have to worry about your body because you know that you're taking care of yourself.

There are some visible signs that you can see to tell that you are dehydrated. These include headaches, chills, dry mouth, dark urine, dizziness, fatigue, and nausea. If you feel any of these symptoms it is recommended that you drink some water immediately. You will soon start to feel better.

Try drinking little sips of water all throughout the day. You will be steadily giving yourself the water and energy you need to do your day-to-day activities and will help you keep yourself healthy for the long-term.

CHAPTER ELEVEN

Balance Your Health

A stool has three legs—just one or two and you fall over. The three primary legs are what you eat, how you exercise, and what happens in your life internally and externally. Never focus on just one—keep a balance.

What we eat determines 70% of our health. With the diet crazes that are constantly sweeping our culture, more and more people are focusing on just reducing their calories, or eating only selected foods. Some diets center on high meat protein, some high carbs, and others focus on blood type or metabolic type. Unbalanced diets like these are narrowly focused on losing weight and have little regard or understanding of basic nutrition.

Limiting our food intake to only what someone else or we believe will help lose weight will never succeed because our bodies become nutritionally unsatisfied. Then our bodies drive us to consume whatever is available to meet our nutritional needs. This is the main reason why diets fail. It isn't just a matter of self-discipline. We must balance our plan with our body's needs.

Try the China Study Diet for a few weeks and see what happens. Reduce your meat and dairy, processed and refined foods, and drink a green smoothie once a day. My basic recipe is on my website. Your body will become nutritionally satisfied; your cravings will diminish and go away. Then work from there. But stay balanced. You'll lose weight down to your ideal weight and stay there naturally.

The second leg, exercise, determines 20% of your health. Get moving, running, hiking, biking, swimming, or any aerobic exercise several times a week. Do some stretching. See my basic stretching routine on the site. Good health requires a good flow of fuel and oxygen to your cells, and removal of waste products. Exercise makes this happen.

Finally, to be truly healthy, the final 10% is our health environment. To stay balanced we need to think, feel, and act positively, both inwardly and outwardly. You have a relationship with yourself and with others that must be nurtured with self-respect and self-esteem. That comes from a sound healthy view of the world, of yourself, and others. Love yourself and enjoy solitary time and love others and enjoy social time with them.

Take time frequently to take your health balance pulse, in all three areas. The study reflects, try out, monitor, and reflect, as you grow in knowledge and health.

Balance Your Health and Life's Goals by Losing Weight Quickly

Life is the name of the game that should be played wisely, magnificently and sometimes ruthlessly. If you do not balance your health and the goals of your life, you will be doing injustice to both of them. If one fades in comparison to your efforts on the other, you cannot call yourself a successful person. Over-weight is the major ingredient for poor health and you should take all possible steps to lose weight quickly so that you can enjoy this magical and wonderful life.

When you decide to lose weight quickly, you should set realistic goals. It is always better to set smaller and achievable goals and succeed in them rather than setting unattainable goals and failing in them because failure may demotivate you. Therefore, you can divide your bigger goal into smaller ones and achieve them slowly and consistently. Setting a big and unattainable goal is one of the major mistakes committed by people while they try to lose weight quickly.

Choice of the foods you eat must be made with utmost caution and care. You should avoid foods that are useless and have no nutritional value such as junk foods, processed foods, spicy and oily foods. These foods cause you more harm than benefits. You cannot lose weight quickly also because they increase your weight to a great extent.

It is better to let all your friends and relatives know that you are on the weight-losing program. This is because whenever they find you trying to over-indulge in a food item that may increase your weight, they may caution you. But you should never seek the opinion of these friends and relatives if you have lost weight. It's unfortunate to know that friends and relatives get jealous faster and more quickly than others who you consider your enemies. These friends and relatives will give you misleading opinions and you may end up making wrong moves in your efforts to lose weight quickly.

Another dangerous thing you may do is to make comparisons of your body with that of others. You should understand that every one of us is different and hence every one of us loses weight at a different rate. You should find out your own methods, foods and other regimens you should follow that suit you the best. No one can impose their prescriptions on you. Of course, you can consult your dietitian or physician who knows your body constitution well and prescribes regimens accordingly.

Instead of taking harmful and useless foods, you can switch to a diet regimen that consists of fiber foods. Fiber foods like green leafy vegetables, fresh fruits, wholesome grains, and beans supply to your body all the essential vitamins and nutrients without increasing your weight. You will also feel the fullness of your stomach more quickly and hence you will not over-eat also. These foods act as a catalyst for you to lose weight quickly.

The above tips will be useful for you to lead a full life so that you can bestow balanced doses of attention on both your health and your life's goals.

The Role of Meditation in Life's Balance

Part of having a balanced life is learning to quiet the mind and focus on issues with a great concentration in order to achieve goals or just to improve the quality of life and enjoy good health.

The ability to focus on the issue at hand is one measure of effectiveness and efficiency. One learns to concentrate and think about one thing at a time. It is hard to think about one thing and nothing else. One of the primary aims of meditation is to tune and train the mind.

There are various exercises that can be practiced as part of the process of mastering meditation or to reach as close to mastery as it is humanly possible to be.

Through our education process, religious leaning or community culture, we accept what is perceived as reality. Often after practicing meditation, we will find that acceptance of things learned while meditating creates a new reality. Meditation changes the perception of the individuals we meet and makes us recognize the humanity in others as well as ourselves.

Learning to meditate is not an easy process. Our minds are usually undisciplined and may refuse to do what we would like to do. There are always many things or events to interrupt our concentration.

We think of other things rather than focus on what we decided to think about.

Meditation may produce a state of deep relaxation, a happier frame of mind as well as a higher alert mental state. Self-improvement and self-empowerment are often the reasons that we undertake to learn meditation in the first place.

Many who suffer from depression, stress and anxiety would benefit from learning and practicing meditation on a regular basis.

Balance your life with meditation and visualization. Practice it daily at a regular time of day or even in the night if you have difficulty sleeping. I often use the all-over-body exercise to get back to sleep if I wake in the night and experience problems falling off to sleep. This exercise allows one to concentrate on each part of the body at a time and to use visualization on each part in a positive, healthy manner. We are what we think. Think positive healthy thoughts, practice meditation, and enjoy good health.

CHAPTER TWELVE

Control Your Anxiety

Anxiety manifests itself in numerous ways depending upon the severity of the disorder. It can begin by worrying about something happening to us or something that we will expect to happen to ourselves, but ultimately the cause of the worry either passes or we learn how to deal with it. Unfortunately, not everyone has the capacity to cope well with what happens in their lives. In fact, there are people who spend almost their entire lives worrying and their worries are part of anxiety symptoms in a never-ending cycle that can produce an anxiety disorder.

Anxiety symptoms can manifest themselves both physically and psychologically. Anxiety disorders happen when our brain warns us about a perceived danger that is about to occur. In this situation, your body will ready itself for a fight or flight reaction. Your heart, lungs and other parts of your body will work faster and produce stress hormones and adrenaline to cope with that time period.

Depending on the perception of the danger, physical symptoms include abdominal discomfort, diarrhea, dry mouth, rapid heartbeat, palpitations, tightness and pain in the chest region, shortness of breath, dizziness, frequent urination and even difficulty swallowing. Such physical effects that anxiety disorders produce can become frightening and enhance the symptoms.

The psychological anxiety symptoms on the other hand include insomnia, irritability, anger, the inability to concentrate on various day to day tasks, a fear of madness, a fear of losing your mind and mental faculties, as well as the sense of being detached from reality and not having the ability to control your actions.

Besides the anxiety symptoms, people may experience emotional symptoms too, such as a constant feeling of unease that has nothing to do with your present situation. Others might experience anxiety due to being involved in a stressful situation like pressure at work or a relationship. Then anxiety symptoms may rear their heads due to being anxious about an illness, real or imagined. Then there is always your body's reaction to perceived dangerous threats. All of these emotional stresses can and will increase the intensity of your anxiety symptoms dramatically.

These symptoms may be considered as anxiety symptoms if they are of a prolonged or severe state, or if the feelings of anxiety come into existence when there is nothing dangerous or stressful to bring them about. Then, if these anxiety symptoms start to interfere with your everyday life and activities like work or social events, you know for certain that you are suffering from an anxiety disorder.

As the world knows, anxiety is a normal response to danger. Everyone has felt anxious about something at some point in their lives. However, there are times when anxiety turns into something else, this being a mental condition known as anxiety disorders. People who have anxiety disorders are sometimes afraid to get treatment for their anxiety as they seem to feel ashamed of having a mental condition. However, anxiety treatments are valid medical remedies for a complaint that can affect your life. There is nothing to be ashamed of having anxiety disorders or being treated for them.

If you might suspect you're suffering from anxiety symptoms, it's always a good idea to get your self-diagnosis confirmed by a qualified medical practitioner who can then start you on the proper course to cure you.

When you first experience anxiety your doctor must be able to diagnose your complaint. There are many types of anxiety treatments that you can try. Before you embark on such a step it's a good idea to talk with a doctor or a psychiatrist who specializes in anxiety and panic disorders. As the treatments can be varied you will need to let your doctor know that you suspect that you are suffering from anxiety disorders so that your specific complaint can be identified. Once your anxiety is diagnosed then treatment may begin.

You might want to ask your doctor what the normal anxiety treatments are and their side effects. You should also find out what their effect will be on your lifestyle as well. Don't rule out alternative remedies—they may not be completely proven by medical science as anxiety treatments, but a number of people state that these alternative treatments can work at providing relief from anxiety symptoms.

The traditional anxiety treatments are prescription drugs like Selective Serotonin Reuptake Inhibitors, Buspirones, anti-depressant medications, and others. These drugs work to lower the chemicals that cause anxiety to surface. While many people have found relief from their anxiety symptoms, these tablets alone may not completely cure your anxiety disorders.

It is like taking an aspirin to relieve a headache, that's all the aspirin does; it does not cure the headache but just reduces the symptoms so that they are bearable.

Alternate anxiety treatments include the age-old methods of Acupuncture and Ayurveda. Both of these eastern anxiety treatments bring the symptoms of anxiety back into control by rebalancing your body's internal energies. These treatments use a number of essential oils, poultices, herbal remedies, and sterilized acupuncture needles to achieve that effect. These alternative anxiety treatments not only control the effects of anxiety in your body they also have the ability to completely cure your anxiety disorder symptoms.

Whatever treatment is decided upon based on advice from your medical practitioner and adviser, by following a course of treatment that works best on your anxiety you stand a good chance of being in control of your life once more and truly at the end that's all that matters.

Types of Anxiety Attacks and Disorders

Having anxiety isn't fun for anyone. At some point, we all experience anxiety, whether under deadline pressure, are scared about something, or just handling a stressful situation. Anxiety is a normal reaction to the stress we all experience in everyday life. Unfortunately, not everyone experiences anxiety the same way. Some people experience anxiety more often and more intensely than the rest of us, perhaps even experiencing anxiety attacks. Too much anxiety can change a person's life and even their feeling of well-being. Millions of adult Americans suffer from some form or type of anxiety disorder. Odds are, you or someone you know or love, is currently being affected by an anxiety disorder.

There are several types of anxiety disorders:

- **Panic Disorders:** Intense anxiety and fears cause unexpected panic or anxiety attacks.

- **Obsessive-Compulsive Disorders:** Performance of consistent or obsessive routines often associated with thoughts or fears that are also considered to be repetitive.

- **Post-Traumatic Stress Disorder (PTSD):** Caused by a traumatic event that leaves a lasting memory of the event.

- **Social Anxiety:** The most common anxiety disorder producing an overwhelming fear and self-consciousness in otherwise normal daily social situations. Social Anxiety is often associated with being afraid of being judged, afraid of making mistakes, being the center of attention, or being fearful of lacking in social skills.

- **Generalized Anxiety Disorder (GAD):** Excessive worrying and tension.

All of these disorders are similar to normal anxiety, except that the level of anxiety rises to the point where constant worry and fear becomes overwhelming.

Anxiety can have very real physical and emotional effects on a person, regardless of how mild the anxiety is. Some of the most common being:

- Neck or back pain
- Headache
- Nausea
- Stomach problems
- Feeling worn out
- Unable to relax
- Weak-feeling muscles
- Unexpected weight loss or gain
- High blood pressure

- Memory loss
- Tired or strained in the eyes

If anxiety is producing any of these physical symptoms in you, it is likely that it is going to affect you mentally and/or emotionally as well. Making matters even worse, these physical effects can even cause additional anxiety.

Having an anxiety attack can be a very terrifying experience. You may have a real problem if you are experiencing them on a regular basis to the point where they:

- Interfere with your work

- Disrupt your family responsibilities or relationships

- Cause avoidance in everyday activities

- And become overwhelming

Symptoms or effects of the anxiety can depend on the level of anxiety or the type of anxiety disorder. The anxiety that escalates into an anxiety attack can be terrifying. They can occur without warning or for any apparent reason. Anxiety attacks can also cause:

- Feelings of losing control
- Chest pain
- Confusion
- Fear
- Muscle tension
- Racing heart
- Difficulty breathing
- Feeling faint
- Nervous shaking
- Dizziness
- Sweating

The physical symptoms of anxiety can resemble a heart attack and be very traumatic. It can often be trigger by the fear of being in a public place or where there may be no help available. Such an attack can also be triggered by just the fear of having another attack.

When anxiety attacks or disorders develop, a person's natural responses are no longer able to deal with the anxiety in healthy ways. The levels of anxiety rise to the point where things become difficult to deal with. It can affect daily situations, ability to perform skills, thought processes and even the physical health of loved ones, acquaintances or even you. Having anxiety can be a serious problem with serious effects and should not be taken lightly or ignored.

Symptoms of Anxiety

We feel anxiety our whole life, even those that don't have the real problem, have experienced anxiety at least 15 minutes a day. When we have an important meeting, and we know that, everything depends on us. There are many common symptoms of Anxiety we go through.

For example, the walls are closing, or maybe we have many debts to pay off, and we just might lose our job if we mess up with the presentation. Some of the common symptoms of anxiety might actually happen in very unthreatening situations such as having a date in the evening. There are many reasons for this, but one is that the problem is in our mind. The good anxieties are the ones when we feel butterflies in our stomach. This is anxiety even though some people decided to name it a bit nicer. So, what are we talking about? Do we all have problems with anxiety?

I am sure that there are at least ten more similar occasions that I can list in order to show you what anxiety is all around, and how it is present in our everyday life. But we have to make a difference between a simple symptom of everyday anxiety that passes during a short period of time and then some that have a more serious anxiety disorder symptoms that are a lot more serious and require the help from the professionals.

The first way you know you are getting into something serious is when you feel scared, and literally freaking out. If you feel like you cannot handle the stress on your own anymore, you must seek professional help. Anxiety disorders develop from too much stress in your life. Whether it's a stressful job or a lot of people depending on you, too much pressure in your life will do that to you. You have to understand that you cannot take care of everything. Something to keep in mind is that anxiety disorders are a lot more serious than your every-day stress and anxiety. There is a major difference is that everyday anxiety might even help you function, but the anxiety disorder does not.

They are followed by some severe problems and symptoms. Usually, the disorder is recognized by the appropriate symptoms and the fact that you are letting anxiety take hold of your life. Symptoms are usually the same for all, but still, some tend to experience some unique symptoms. Here are some of the most common anxiety symptoms, ones that you can look for.

Emotional symptoms are a bit tricky since you can have these symptoms in common situations. But remember, if it crosses the border of normal everyday stress only then can it be considered an anxiety disorder. Feelings of apprehension or dread, trouble with concentrating, feeling tense and jumpy, always anticipating the worst, feeling of restlessness, constantly watching for the signs of danger and the feeling that your mind has gone blank. Usually, these emotional symptoms take hold of your everyday life activities, in so much an extent that you no longer worry about anything but only of your feelings, worries, and fear. To sum things, the top three most common anxiety disorders are; constant worry, fear, and unemotional stress. In addition, some most common physical symptoms are the pounding of your heart, sweating, stomach upset or dizziness, frequent urination or diarrhea, shortness of breath, tremors and twitches, muscle tension, headaches, insomnia are the most common symptoms that your body produces as a response to your emotions.

Again, I have to underline that there is a difference between anxiety and anxiety disorder. Anxiety disorders prevent you from leading a normal life, whatever normal may mean to you. The anxiety disorder is treatable in 100 % of all people that suffer from it, so don't ignore them, better try to solve them. And basically, these most common symptoms of Anxiety will not let you lead a normal life.

There are some simple explanations of anxiety symptoms:

EMOTIONAL SYMPTOMS:

- Irritability.
- Lack of concentration.
- Tension.
- Restlessness.
- Foreseeing the worst.
- Looking for danger signs.
- Having a blank mind.
- Feeling of nearing death or apprehension.

PHYSICAL SYMPTOMS:

- Excessive perspiration.
- Pounding heart.
- Dizziness and Nausea.
- Diarrhea.

- Frequent urination.
- Breathlessness.
- Tremors.
- Headaches.
- Insomnia or sleeplessness.

- Muscle tension.
- Chest pain.
- Choking sensation.
- Hyperventilation.
- Chills or hot flashes.

If you have been experiencing any of these symptoms of anxiety attacks, please visit your doctor without further delay. Anxiety attacks can be prevented and the faster you realize that, the better for you.

Treatment of Anxiety

When looking for a treatment for anxiety disorder there are various options available for you, but which treatment do you choose?

Anxiety disorder symptoms can vary and they can make you feel anxious and helpless most of the time without any logical reason. These feelings can be very frightening and they may lead people to even stop doing what they really enjoy for fear of an attack.

Depending on how severe your circumstances may be has a huge bearing on the choices of treatment available to you. You need to be guided by your doctor who will assess the extent of your condition and then recommend treatment from there.

DIAGNOSIS AND TREATMENT FOR ANXIETY DISORDER

In many cases, symptoms of anxiety disorders can get masked by various medical conditions, which can make their diagnosis quite difficult. Quite often, an episode is accompanied by depression and in many cases, symptoms may overlap. A thorough examination by your GP can help in eliminating any medical issues. Once the disorder is successfully identified, a treatment plan can be recommended by using medication, or psychiatric therapy, or in some cases, a combination of alternative and standard therapies can be used to get the desired results.

TREATMENT USING MEDICATION

In most cases, medication is used in conjunction with other therapies, or alternative forms of anxiety treatment. Sometimes medicines are used alone depending upon the condition of the patient and his or her preference of treatment. Though medication alone, when used for the treatment for anxiety disorder, may not be the cure for this condition, it can be used by patients to keep the disorder under control. Often medication goes hand in hand with another method too.

When medication is prescribed for treating this disorder, doctors first try to diagnose any contributing causes that may interfere with the performance of medication. As many patients of anxiety disorders are also affected by some substance abuse or depression, a doctor may even suggest separate treatment for these problems.

DRUGS USED IN THE TREATMENT OF THE DISORDER

Depending upon the intensity and symptoms shown, doctors can prescribe medications from amongst three categories of drugs:

- Beta blockers

- Anti-anxiety drugs

- Anti-depressants

Quite often a lot of doctors rely on anti-depressants as they are highly effective in treating anxiety disorders where patients are also diagnosed with depression.

All those who have a joint diagnosis with alcohol or drug abuse may also be giving benzodiazepines. The problem here is one of dependency as a lot of these types of drugs are addictive, so they are only given for a short time.

Beta blockers such as propranolol that are used for treating various heart ailments are also prescribed for the treatment of anxiety disorder.

NATURAL TREATMENTS FOR ANXIETY

Natural treatments for anxiety do exist and it isn't always necessary to go on medication. There are a couple of alternatives to medication that you can try to help treat and hopefully eliminate your anxiety attacks.

Herbs

Natural treatments like passionflower and Kava have shown to decrease anxiety as equivalent to taking benzodiazepine drugs; however, caution should still be taken even with herbs as many may have side effects as well. Side effects of passionflower can include nausea, vomiting, drowsiness, and rapid heartbeat. Kava and passionflower tea can be a great way to try these herbs as a tea which often causes fewer problems than taking the dietary supplements. If you suffer from mild anxiety, you may find improvement with the herb Valerian; its strengths are in helping with insomnia.

Massage

When you suffer from chronic anxiety your body never relaxes; this can have serious side effects on it is own leading to headaches, jaw pain, difficulty falling and/or staying asleep, muscle tension and more. Using massage therapy or shiatsu to treat your anxiety can help address all of these issues, it can help loosen your muscles, calm your mind and ultimately put you at ease. With improved sleep and being in a relaxed state, you may notice that your anxiety slowly decreases over time.

CHAPTER THIRTEEN

Cultivate Healthy Relationships

At the breakup of a relationship, most of the time you feel like giving up. Many people drown their sorrows in drink or drugs or even a combination of both. Some look for ex-quotes to soothe their hearts and many women rush for ex-boyfriend quotes. Is this a good thing? Maybe not.

The simplest way you can uplift yourself is by taking time to relax. Often, individuals end up with depressive disorders or even anxiety as they're overloaded. If you take possibly one hour out of your day just to relax, read through a novel or watch television, your body and mind are steadier to handle crucial issues.

Avoid worrying a great deal about yourself. That might seem counter-intuitive, but when you start off watching what you can do for other people as opposed to worrying about yourself a lot, good things can happen. Often the thankfulness of others when you've done self-less acts is merely frosting on the cake and you will then boost the way you see yourself as well.

Another thing you can consider when you are looking to improve yourself, your job, as well as your points of view and outlooks about life, is to live life on your own! Do not take into account that which folks may want you to do, talk or behave, as this stops your individual development at a lot of important stages.

Beat your personal worries with action. Use baby steps in order to overcome your own doubts either to lessen their particular grip on you or even to entirely get rid of them. Convince yourself you could become more than simply afraid of the fears, and that you may take actions to avoid them all. Don't be restricted by them.

Never allow putting things off to keep you from achieving your objectives. It's always too simple to find why you should put off making the first step towards achieving success. Also, the more you delay, the more difficult it will be, to be determined. The reality is, should you start right now, you are going to easily build up energy, helping you to accomplish your own desired goals faster than you ever imagined achievable.

Recognize all your faults as well as errors. Don't avoid any of them for the sake of positivity. Strong-willed absurdity may weaken you more than any sort of flaw or even oversight ever could. The beneficial change will come out of analyzing all your disadvantages and changing them into places where you can learn and grow. People today admire and have confidence in a person that will acknowledge whenever they've done wrong.

Make an effort to learn to breathe properly. You should be in a position to concentrate on your inhaling and exhaling, especially if you are stressed or perhaps in some sort of discomfort. As soon as tasks get intensive, stay away from taking rapid breaths that can make you dizzy and even pass out, as an alternative try to inhale and exhale slowly and deeply. You can easily really feel a lot more in control of your anxiety as well as pain to prevent making things more serious.

Regularly following this regiment will take you a long way in overcoming a breakup or some other personal crisis and will do more good than ex-boyfriend quotes or other quotes ever will.

Our life revolves around three basic things:

- Physical health

- Professional life

- Relationships

I call them circles of concern and these circles will inevitably overlap each other. Financial worries will affect your relationships and your relationship has a direct influence on your business life. It is impossible to live in one circle and forget about the other one.

Your physical health has the same importance. When you are sick you cannot perform well. You cannot enjoy life without enjoying sound health.

Every relationship is important. The two most important relationships are:

- Your relationship with your spouse

- Your relationship with your children

Every one of us goes through two major decisions of our life:

- Choice of life partner

- Choice of a good career

We have to make these decisions while we are teenagers. It is good to decide your career before you are 18 because a good career is a path to financial prosperity and happiness. Advise your son and daughter to choose their career before they graduate from college.

Relationships become critical when your age is between 40 to 50 years. This is the most productive time of your life. You are mature and you are on the hot seat of decisions.

Also, this is the most responsible stage of your life. Business problems are there and you have to take care of your teenage children. This is the time when you will reap what you have sown.

Problems occur when your relationships are not good with your spouse and children. Teenagers want to express themselves. It is a critical time. They are not fully mature and they are emotional. It is your job to understand their emotions and talents.

As parents, only you can understand them better. They need your love and understanding. Just like a financial bank account, there is a financial bank account. If you will not deposit kind deeds in your emotional bank account, it will remain empty and you will be bankrupt. Most people face that bankruptcy when they are in their 40s. Their teenage son is not doing well and parents are blaming each other for the cause.

In my opinion, this is the basic problem and that is why your health goes down. Your home should be a peaceful place for you with your spouse and children. Life is a journey. The difficult time comes and goes. A good relationship will always help you in crisis, whether you face financial problems or health issues.

Conclusion

In conclusion, new habits can be established in a matter of weeks. It takes a very short time to change from old, ineffective ways of living and introduce better, more constructive personal habits, improved confidence and self-esteem results in a healthier and more satisfying lifestyle. A positive work, family and personal life generates less stress. This is indeed a worthwhile outcome from the changes.

Bibliography

Colberg, S. R., Sigal, R. J., Fernhall, B., Regensteiner, J. G., Blissmer, B., Rubin, R. R.,…Braun, B. (2010). Exercise and Type 2 Diabetes: The American College of Sports Medicine and the American Diabetes Association: Joint Position Statement Executive Summary. *Diabetes Care, 33*(12), 2692-2696. Retrieved 12 27, 2019, from https://ncbi.nlm.nih.gov/pmc/articles/pmc2992214

Thompson, P. D., Buchner, D., Piña, I. L., Balady, G. J., Williams, M. A., Marcus, B. H.,… Wenger, N. K. (2003). Exercise and Physical Activity in the Prevention and Treatment of Atherosclerotic Cardiovascular Disease A Statement From the Council on Clinical Cardiology (Subcommittee on Exercise, Rehabilitation, and Prevention) and the Council on Nutrition, Physical Activity, and Metabolism (Subcommittee on Physical Activity). *Circulation, 107*(24), 3109 -3116. Retrieved 12 27, 2019, from https://ahajournals.org/doi/10.1161/01 .cir.0000075572.40158.77